Medical Mathematics and Dosage Calculations
for Veterinary Technicians

Medical Mathematics and Dosage Calculations for Veterinary Technicians

Third Edition

Robert Bill
Professor Emeritus
College of Veterinary Medicine
Purdue University
West Lafayette, Indiana, USA

WILEY Blackwell

Edition History
Iowa State University Press (1e, 2000); Wiley-Blackwell (2e, 2009)

Registered Office(s)
John Wiley & Sons, Inc., 111 River Street, Hoboken, NJ 07030, USA

Editorial Office
111 River Street, Hoboken, NJ 07030, USA

For details of our global editorial offices, customer services, and more information about Wiley products visit us at www.wiley.com.

Wiley also publishes its books in a variety of electronic formats and by print-on-demand. Some content that appears in standard print versions of this book may not be available in other formats.

Library of Congress Cataloging-in-Publication Data

Names: Bill, Robert, author.
Title: Medical mathematics and dosage calculations for veterinary technicians / Robert Bill.
Other titles: Medical mathematics and dosage calculations for veterinary professionals
Description: 3rd edition. | Hoboken, NJ : John Wiley & Sons, Inc., 2019. | Includes index. |
    Preceded by Medical mathematics and dosage calculations for veterinary professionals /
    Robert Bill. 2nd ed. 2009. |
Identifiers: LCCN 2018032830 (print) | LCCN 2018033237 (ebook) | ISBN 9781118924136 (Adobe PDF) |
    ISBN 9781118924143 (ePub) | ISBN 9781118835296 (pbk.)
Subjects: | MESH: Veterinary Drugs–administration & dosage | Drug Dosage Calculations |
    Mathematics | Handbooks
Classification: LCC SF917 (ebook) | LCC SF917 (print) | NLM SF 919 | DDC 636.089/51–dc23
LC record available at https://lccn.loc.gov/2018032830

Cover Design: Wiley
Cover Images: © DenGuy/E+/Getty Images; © aydinmutlu/E+/Getty Images; © SchulteProductions/E+/Getty Images

Set in 10/12pt Warnock by SPi Global, Pondicherry, India

SKY10079405_071124

Contents

About the Companion Website

This book is accompanied by a companion website:

www.wiley.com/go/bill/calculations

The website includes:
- Answer keys to problems
- PowerPoint files of all figures from the book for downloading

Section I

Review of Math Fundamentals

1

Math Fundamentals

Self-assessment

OBJECTIVES
The student will be able to: 1) conduct a self-assessment, and 2) identify areas needed for review.

In a medical situation the most beneficial drug can be rendered worthless or dangerous if the veterinarian or veterinary technician does not accurately calculate the dose. As many veterinary professionals can testify, it is not enough to just have a superficial understanding of dosage calculation because superficial knowledge often fails during an emergency situation. The skill of accurately calculating drug dosages or making correct medical math calculations must be deeply ingrained and practiced to be consistently reliable.

Another obligation of professionals is to recognize and accurately identify the limits of their knowledge and to strengthen the weaker areas of their skills or knowledge. To help you define the areas of math and dosage calculation that you need to refresh or review, complete the following self-assessment exercises. Note that some of the exercises require you to perform the tasks *without a calculator*. Although a calculator should be used to carry out most dosage calculations, it is also important that the veterinary professional understands how to perform the basic operations manually. They will thereby be able to recognize when an answer to a problem is obviously not accurate (e.g. when the decimal point is misplaced by 1 or 2 places).

For those sections of the self-assessment that you identify as areas where a review would be useful, work through the chapters and sections of the book to which that section of the self-assessment exercise refers.

Self-assessment Exercises

1 Write each of the following numbers in scientific notation:

   A) 23
   B) 132
   C) 522 178
   D) 0.2
   E) 0.0452

Medical Mathematics and Dosage Calculations for Veterinary Technicians, Third Edition. Robert Bill.
© 2019 John Wiley & Sons, Inc. Published 2019 by John Wiley & Sons, Inc.
Companion website: www.wiley.com/go/bill/calculations

F) 0.000 067

G) 94.0023

H) 897.010 00

2 Add or subtract the following decimal numbers, without a calculator:

A) $1.5 + 4 =$

B) $9.7 + 1.9 =$

C) $6.55 + 7.43 =$

D) $0.42 + 0.09 =$

E) $0.009 + 4.0 =$

F) $7.5 - 2.5 =$

G) $9.0 - 3.9 =$

H) $23.125 - 1.50 =$

I) $0.551 - 0.095 =$

J) $0.003 52 - 0.0009 =$

K) The veterinarian needs a mixture of the following three drugs to be administered as an anesthetic cocktail: 0.4 mL Drug A, 0.35 mL Drug B, and 1.24 mL of Drug C. What is the final volume of combined drug to be given?

L) Four gerbils are weighed individually. Their masses are 82.0 g, 76.5 g, 92.8 g, and 81.9 g. What is the total weight of all four gerbils?

M) The normal dose for an animal is calculated as 48.7 mg. However, the veterinarian wants to adjust the dose because of changes in the animal's physiology due to the disease being treated. The dose needs to be decreased by 10% (4.87 mg). What is the new dose need for this patient?

N) The veterinarian gives an oral drug order to be added to a bag of IV fluids as follows: "Give twenty-three point four mL of Drug A and three point one two five mL of Drug B." What is the total volume (mL) of drugs being added to this bag of IV fluids?

3 Multiply or divide the following decimal numbers, without a calculator:

A) $2.5 \times 5 =$

B) $3.0 \times 8.35 =$

C) $24.75 \times 12.35 =$

D) $0.02 \times 15.5 =$

E) $0.003 \times 0.0125 =$

F) $15 \div 2.5 =$

G) $2.5 \div 1.5 =$

H) $35 \div 0.5 =$

I) $0.25 \div 0.125 =$

J) $0.010 \div 0.0025 =$

K) An animal is dispensed 2.5 mg tablets to be given twice daily for six days. What is the total mass of drug that has been dispensed? Give your answer in mg.

L) The veterinarian dispenses 1200 mL of medication to be given equally to 8 calves. How much does each calf get?

M) A laboratory animal colony needs to treat a parasite problem by giving 2.3 mg of a drug to each of the 94 rats in the colony. How many mg of drug is needed to do this?

N) A total of 560 mg of drug needs to be equally divided into two doses per day for a period of one week. How much drug is given in each dose?

O) The veterinarian gives the following drug order: "Dispense one and one-tenth mL per day for ten days." What total volume (mL) is to be dispensed?

P) A veterinarian gives the following oral drug order: "42.75 mL of drug needs to be divided into equal doses for these three cats." How much does each cat get?

4 Round the following decimal numbers to the nearest 1/100th and the nearest 1/10th, without a calculator:

A) 20.394 =

B) 9.682 =

C) 3.233 =

D) 29.452 =

E) 413.675 =

F) 5.956 =

G) 36.789 22 =

H) 0.255 =

I) 0.093 =

J) 1200.019 22 =

K) The veterinarian gives the following oral drug order: "Give fifteen point seven five mg but round it to the nearest tenth." How much do you give?

L) The dose calculation for a patient is 37.56 mg. What would the dose be, correctly rounded to a whole number? Is this dose closer to the 40 mg tablet size or the 35 mg tablet size?

5 Simplify the following fractions to their lowest form (e.g. 6/8 = 3/4), without a calculator:

A) $\dfrac{2}{10} =$

B) $\dfrac{4}{16} =$

C) $\dfrac{3}{12} =$

D) $1\dfrac{6}{8} =$

E) $5\dfrac{4}{32} =$

6 Add or subtract the following fractions, without a calculator:

A) $\dfrac{1}{4} + \dfrac{3}{4} =$

B) $\dfrac{1}{16} + \dfrac{3}{32} =$

C) $\dfrac{1}{6} + \dfrac{2}{5} =$

D) $1\dfrac{3}{4} + 2\dfrac{1}{2} =$

E) $5\dfrac{2}{3} + 4\dfrac{7}{8} =$

F) $\dfrac{1}{2} - \dfrac{1}{4} =$

G) $\dfrac{2}{3} - \dfrac{1}{6} =$

H) $1\dfrac{3}{4} - \dfrac{7}{8} =$

I) $3\dfrac{15}{16} - 2\dfrac{3}{8} =$

J) $45\dfrac{1}{5} - 33\dfrac{7}{8} =$

7 Multiply the following fractions, without a calculator:

A) $\dfrac{1}{2} \times \dfrac{1}{2} =$

B) $\dfrac{3}{4} \times \dfrac{1}{2} =$

C) $\dfrac{12}{16} \times \dfrac{3}{4} =$

D) $1\dfrac{1}{2} \times \dfrac{7}{8} =$

E) $\dfrac{11}{16} \times \dfrac{3}{4} =$

F) $2\dfrac{3}{4} \times 4\dfrac{1}{2} =$

G) $5\dfrac{4}{7} \times 1\dfrac{3}{4} =$

H) $10\dfrac{3}{8} \times 9\dfrac{1}{3} =$

8 Divide the following fractions:

A) $\dfrac{1}{4} \div \dfrac{1}{2} =$

B) $\dfrac{1}{3} \div \dfrac{1}{2} =$

C) $\dfrac{2}{4} \div \dfrac{3}{9} =$

D) $2 \div \dfrac{1}{4} =$

E) $2\frac{1}{2} \div \frac{1}{2} =$

F) $3\frac{3}{4} \div \frac{1}{16} =$

G) $22\frac{4}{8} \div \frac{2}{32} =$

H) $125\frac{1}{5} \div \frac{4}{25} =$

9   Convert the following fractions to decimal numbers (e.g. 1/2 = 0.5):

A) $\frac{2}{10} =$

B) $\frac{14}{28} =$

C) $\frac{3}{21} =$

D) $1\frac{1}{2} =$

E) $4\frac{5}{6} =$

F) $15\frac{7}{16} =$

10   Convert the following decimal numbers to the common fraction (e.g. 0.5 = 1/2):

A) 0.25 =
B) 0.333 =
C) 0.75 =
D) 0.125 =
E) 1.5 =
F) 2.500 =

11   Convert the following percentages to commonly used fractions (e.g. 50% = 1/2):

A) 25% =
B) 75% =
C) 33.3% =
D) 10% =
E) 80% =

12   Convert the following percentages to decimal numbers:

A) 25% =
B) 79% =

C) 100% =

D) 6% =

E) 0.2% =

F) 0.0087% =

13 Convert the following decimal numbers to percentages:

A) 0.5 =

B) 0.45 =

C) 1.00 =

D) 0.103 =

E) 0.900 23 =

14 Convert the following fractions to percentages (e.g. 1/2 = 50%):

A) $\dfrac{3}{4}$ =

B) $\dfrac{8}{10}$ =

C) $\dfrac{15}{45}$ =

D) $\dfrac{10}{10}$ =

E) $\dfrac{1}{1000}$ =

15 Answer the following percentage questions:

A) What is 25% of a 200 mg dose?

B) A veterinarian wants to use 50% of 25 mg calculated dose. How much drug (in milligrams) would they be giving?

C) What percentage is 80 pounds of 400 pounds?

D) A veterinary technician has drawn up 15 mg of the total 60 mg drug dose that they need to give an animal. What percentage of the total dose have they drawn up so far?

16 Solve for the missing X in each of the following:

A) $15 + X = 30 + 45$

B) $5 + 10 = 7 + X$

C) $X + 2.5 = 5.25 + 1.05$

D) $40 - X = 65 - 38$

E) $6.5 - 2.3 = 7.8 - X$

F) $X - 14.2 = 53.4 - 41.9$

17 Solve for the missing X in each of the following:

A) $2 \times 6 = 3 \times X$

B) $30 \times X = 120 \times 2$

C) $X \times 25.5 = 43.2 \times 12.25$
D) $25 \div 5 = 10 \div X$
E) $300 \div X = 12.5 \div 8.125$
F) $X \div 25 = 0.5 \div 0.75$

18 Solve for the missing X in the following proportions:

A) $\dfrac{2}{8} = \dfrac{X}{16}$

B) $\dfrac{4}{16} = \dfrac{3}{X}$

C) $\dfrac{X}{32} = \dfrac{18}{9}$

D) $\dfrac{12}{2} = \dfrac{X}{6}$

E) $\dfrac{9}{X} = \dfrac{36}{12}$

2

Review of Key Medical Math Fundamentals

Decimals

OBJECTIVES

The student will be able to:

1) accurately communicate decimal numbers in writing and speaking,
2) add and subtract decimals,
3) multiply and divide decimals,
4) apply scientific notation, and
5) round numbers.

Drug dosages, concentrations of drugs in vials, and drug units are commonly expressed as decimal numbers. Therefore, it is imperative that the veterinary professional be able to accurately add, subtract, multiply, and divide using decimal numbers. It is assumed the reader has a working knowledge of using decimals; therefore, this chapter will focus on a quick review with an emphasis on where common dosage calculation errors occur.

2.1 Relative Values of Decimal Numbers

The decimal point, or "point," orients the reader to the values of the decimal number. Each space to the *left* of the decimal point increases by a power of 10. Therefore, the first space to the left of the decimal point is "ones," the next space to the left is "tens," the next is "hundreds," and so on.

Each space to the *right* of the decimal point decreases by a power of 10 starting with "tenths." The second space to the right of the decimal point is the "hundredths," the next is "thousandths," and so on. Note that there are no "oneths" to the right of the decimal point and the first place to the right starts with "tenths." The numerals to the left of the decimal point are *whole numbers* (5, 62, 379) and the numerals to the right of the decimal point represent *decimal fractions* (e.g. one tenth, four hundredths).

Notice how all decimal fractions end in "th(s)," such as "four ten*ths*" or "one thousand*th*." Thus, the number 12.35 would contain the whole number "12" and the decimal fraction of "thirty-five hundredths."

The number shown in Figure 2.1 is 7842.125 and illustrates each of the places in the number.

Medical Mathematics and Dosage Calculations for Veterinary Technicians, Third Edition. Robert Bill.
© 2019 John Wiley & Sons, Inc. Published 2019 by John Wiley & Sons, Inc.
Companion website: www.wiley.com/go/bill/calculations

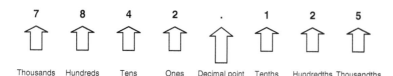

				.			
7	8	4	2		1	2	5
⇧	⇧	⇧	⇧	⇧	⇧	⇧	⇧
Thousands	Hundreds	Tens	Ones	Decimal point	Tenths	Hundredths	Thousandths

Whole numbers   **Decimal fractions**

Figure 2.1 The location of whole numbers and decimal fractions in a decimal number

2.2 Properly Communicating Decimal Numbers

When reading a decimal number aloud, there are two ways to communicate the number. The number in Figure 2.1 can be read as either "seven thousand, eight hundred forty-two and one hundred twenty-five thousandths" or as "seven eight four two point one two five."

The first method is more formal and uses the word "and" to represent the decimal point. All units to the right of the decimal point are read as units of the *farthest right* place. Therefore, in the number above, there are "125 thousandths." For the number "1.12," the value to the right of the decimal point would be read aloud as "twelve hundredths" because the farthest right place that has a number is the hundredths place. When the value of a decimal number is less than 1, such as 0.5, the number would be read only as "five tenths" without stating the zero in the ones place.

The second method for communicating decimal numbers tends to convey the information in a shorter and more concise manner. The numbers are read left to right with the decimal point being spoken as "point." No place values (hundreds, tenths, thousandths, etc.) are stated in this method. Therefore, "234.56" would simply be read aloud as "two three four point five six." In contrast to the first method above, where the zero is not read for numbers with a value less than 1, in this second method the zero is communicated along with the "point." Thus 0.5 would be read as "zero point five." There are additional examples in Table 2.1.

Regardless of which method is used when a number is verbally communicated, it is essential that the number be communicated accurately. This can be a challenge when numbers are being communicated while masked for surgery or other procedures because the voice becomes muffled. It also becomes a challenge when communicating numbers by phone, particularly as cell phone reception can garble clear communication. In addition to the physical challenges with communicating numbers, some numbers sounds very similar to others, and the veterinary technician needs to be especially precise in communicating these numbers. It is a good practice to repeat any number that may be confusing, or to emphasize a key feature of the number, such as "One five POINT three," to make sure the recipient correctly receives the number. If there

Table 2.1 The correct way to read decimal numbers

36.89	"Thirty-six and eighty-nine hundredths" "Three six point eight nine"
0.9	"Nine tenths" "Zero point nine"
0.076	"Seventy-six thousandths" "Zero point zero seven six"
30.08	"Thirty and eight hundredths" "Three zero point zero eight"

is *ever* a question about what number was stated by another staff member or the veterinarian, the veterinary technician is ethically and morally obligated to ask that the number be repeated. Reluctance to ask because of perceived irritation or frustration of the person stating the number is absolutely no reason not to be crystal clear on what number was being communicated. The veterinary technician is the advocate for the patient, and therefore it is essential all numeric communications be accurately communicated 100% of the time.

Commonly miscommunicated numbers

There are several numbers that, when read, sound very similar. It is important that the veterinary professional clearly enunciate these to prevent accidental miscommunication of a spoken value. It is also important that, if any question arises of what value is being communicated, the receiver of the spoken value ask for the value to be repeated. A patient's life could hang in the balance.

- Thirteen sounds like thirty.

- Fourteen sounds like forty.

- Fifteen sounds like fifty.

- Sixteen sounds like sixty.

- Seventeen sounds like seventy.

- Eighteen sounds like eighty.

- Nineteen sounds like ninety.

While all of the decimal fractions sound like their counterpart in the whole numbers (e.g. "tenth" and "ten," "hundredth" and "hundred"), generally, the context in which the number is spoken prevents it from being confused (e.g. "three hundred and twenty-three hundredths" for the number 300.23). If there is any doubt, however, the number needs to be repeated to confirm all parties understand the actual number communicated.

2.3   The Rules for the Use of Zero in Decimal Numbers

Rule 1: Whole numbers (e.g. 2, 45, 789) have implied decimal points and trailing zeroes to the right of the decimal point that are usually not written or spoken. "25" and "25.00" both represent the same value of 25 and therefore would be communicated as "twenty-five" unless greater precision is required. For example, a patient's blood chemistry value may always be printed out or displayed on the laboratory equipment with a number in the 1/10ths slot. In those situations, "25.0" would be communicated as "twenty-five point zero" or "two five point zero" to emphasize that there is no other number in the 1/10ths slot. Another example may be that a dose of a toxic drug is required to be calculated to the nearest 1/10th. In that situation the digit in the 1/10th slot would always be written or communicated, even if the digit was zero.

Another reason for leaving off the trailing zeros is because the decimal point could potentially be mistaken as a comma. For example, at quick glance, the numbers "25.000" and "25,000" look very similar, especially if the numbers are handwritten by a doctor or a veterinary technician in a hurry. A mistake made by not correctly interpreting the comma or decimal point can result in a dose miscalculation of a thousand times more than what was intended! To avoid this problem with handwritten numbers, commas should not to be used in written calculations.

In our global economy it is important to remember that a comma is used in place of the decimal point in many non-English speaking countries in continental Europe and Latin America (except Mexico) and also in South Africa. In these countries the decimal point is used like the comma to separate the digits in large numbers and the comma is used to separate the ones from the 1/10ths in the number. Thus, one may see "2.64 mg" written as "2,64 mg" in France, Germany, Austria, and many other countries around the world. The period as the decimal separator is used predominantly in North America (with the exception of French-speaking Canada) and in the UK, Australia, and other countries where English is commonly used in business or medical communications. In the UK, the "period" is also referred to as a "full stop." To avoid this confusion in countries where either decimal point system may be used, large value numbers are sometimes written as groups of three digits separated from each other by a space instead of a comma or period between thousands and millions. Thus, "one million three hundred thousand" would look like "1 300 000" with spaces but no delimiters between the three digit groups.

This text will use the decimal convention with no comma delimiters, in keeping with generally accepted practices in most of North America, but the veterinary professional needs to be aware of the possible variations of the decimal-delimiter format used in countries worldwide.

Rule 2: Zeros between the decimal point and any integer (1, 2, 5, etc.) to the right of the decimal point are always written and spoken.

For example, "one and three hundredths" would be written as "1.03," and "forty-three thousandths" would be written as "0.043." The number "1.03" could be spoken as "one and three hundredths," but would probably be better and more accurately spoken as "one point zero three" to remove the need for someone having to translate where the "three hundredths" would be placed in the written decimal number.

Rule 3: If a decimal number has a value of less than one, a zero should always be put in the ones place to call attention to the decimal point. The numbers "5" and ".5" can look alike if read quickly or if they are handwritten and the decimal point is not clearly written. Failure to note the decimal point could potentially result in a 10× overdose of the drug. So, instead of writing ".5," the veterinary professional should always write "0.5" with a zero in the ones place to call attention to the presence of the decimal point. When communicating the number 0.543, it would be best to state it as "zero point five four three". "Five hundred and forty-three thousandths" could be interpreted as either 0.543 or 500.043.

2.4 Comparing Decimals – Which Number Is Larger?

Errors sometimes occur in performing changes of doses for a patient because the mind does not recognize that a decimal number with a smaller value may actually look like a decimal number with a larger value. For example, at first glance the mind may interpret the value of 0.095 as being larger than 0.1 when it is not. After all, "ninety-five" is much larger than "one." To catch calculation accidents where there has been an inappropriately placed decimal, and to also provide the veterinary professional with a means of quickly checking the validity of their calculated answer, it is important to gain a "feel" for the relative size of decimal numbers.

Here is an example of where an appreciation for the relative size of decimal numbers could prevent a mistake. A drug has a listed acceptable dose range of 0.125–0.2 mg (an acceptable dose is anything inside of this dose range). The dose the veterinary technician just calculated for this sized patient came out to 0.36 mg of drug. Just by looking at the calculated value and the acceptable dose range, is this calculated dose appropriate?

Without thinking properly, a part of the veterinary technician's brain might think that the required dose range for this drug is between "2 and 125," the calculated value of "36" is in the middle of this range, and therefore the dose makes sense to give. However, administering this dose would result in an overdose and a potentially toxic response because the dose is not within the acceptable range of possible doses.

An easy way to prevent drawing this inaccurate conclusion is to add trailing zeroes to all of the values so the numbers are all filled out to the same number of slots to the right of the decimal point. Writing 0.2 mg as 0.200 mg and 0.36 as 0.360 does nothing to change the actual value of the number, but it makes it easier to compare decimal numbers and to more readily see how the numbers compare to each other. Now the eye and brain can more readily see that the acceptable range (as whole numbers) is "125–200" and the value calculated of "360" is too high a dose. The dose must be lowered to prevent harming the patient.

2.5 A Quick Guide to Using Scientific Notation

Look at these numbers:

1000000, 10000000, 1000000, 1000000, 1000000

Were they all the same number? Is there one that is different from the rest? By carefully examining each number, you should see that one number is ten times larger than the rest. However, this exercise illustrates how easy it is for the brain to confuse large numbers when they are written out.

To reduce confusion with using numbers that have very large or very small values, such decimal or whole numbers are often expressed in "scientific notation." Scientific notation is sometimes also called "exponential notation" because of the use of the exponent (10^x) in the expression. Scientific notation expresses a numerical value as some number multiplied to a "power of 10." Below are several numbers expressed in scientific notation. Can you identify the pattern for how scientific notation works?

$$10 = 1 \times 10^1$$
$$100 = 1 \times 10^2$$
$$20 = 2 \times 10^1$$
$$2000 = 2 \times 10^3$$
$$2500 = 2.5 \times 10^3$$
$$2530 = 2.53 \times 10^3$$
$$253\,000\,000 = 2.53 \times 10^8$$

Scientific notation is written with five elements to more concisely represent much larger numbers:

1) a single integer placed to the left of the decimal point;
2) a decimal point following the single integer;
3) any other integers from the number placed to the right of the decimal point (the "significant numbers");

4) a "times" symbol ("×") indicating the decimal is to be multiplied; and

5) the value of 10 (called the "base") raised to the appropriate multiple of 10 ($100 = 10^2$, $1000 = 10^3$, $10\,000 = 10^4$, etc.) expressed by the superscripted number (the "exponent").

Examples of numbers converted to their correct scientific notation are shown in Table 2.2.

Table 2.2 Examples of numbers converted to scientific notation.

Original number	Scientific notation
55	5.5×10^1
465	4.65×10^2
15 362	1.5362×10^4
30	3×10^1
509	5.09×10^2
9	9×10^0
0.8	8×10^{-1}
0.043	4.3×10^{-2}
0.000 67	6.7×10^{-4}
0.010 20	1.02×10^{-2}
291.365	$2.913\,65 \times 10^2$
4500.90	4.5009×10^3

To convert a number such as 4000 to scientific notation, the integer in the largest place value (in this case "4" in the thousands slot) is written as a decimal number with a period ("4.") and the remainder of the original number is placed to the right of the decimal ("4.000"). This number is then multiplied by 10 raised to the value of the original number. The original number was a thousand (4000), so the exponent to which the base 10 would be raised would be 3, giving "$\times 10^3$" (because $10 \times 10 \times 10 = 1000$). Another way of determining the exponent number is to count how many places the decimal point was moved to go from the original number to the scientific notation number (e.g. to go from 4000 to 4.000 required the decimal point to be moved three places, so the exponent becomes three: 10^3).

To simplify reading scientific notation once the conversion to scientific notation is completed, the trailing zeroes to the right of the decimal point can be deleted. If there are no integers remaining to the right of the decimal point after the trailing zeroes have been removed, the decimal point itself can be removed ("3.000" becomes "3").

Note that 10^1 is base 10 raised one time and is equal to "10." So the expression "3×10^1" is the same as to "3×10" or 30. Because the use of the superscripted "1" exponent is redundant, 10^1 is typically not used for scientific convention (however, if a number is to be written in scientific notation, it should be included since the exponent is a component of true scientific notation). Note also that 10^0 is the same value as 1, therefore the number written scientifically as "4.5×10^0" would be the same value as "4.5×1" or 4.5. Again the 10^0 is typically not used in medical communication using the scientific notation.

To convert scientific notation back to a decimal number, just remove the 10 and exponent, and move the decimal point to the right the number of times equal to the value of the exponent. For example, to convert the number expressed in scientific notation as 5.431×10^3 to its decimal number equivalent would require moving the decimal point in 5.431 three places to the *right* because 10 is raised to the power of 3. Moving the decimal point three places to the *right* gives the original number of 5431.

For decimal numbers with values less than 1, the basic rules for writing scientific notation rules still apply, but the exponent superscript consists of negative numbers (–1, –2, –3, etc.) instead of positive numbers. The negative numbers indicate that the decimal point is moving in the opposite direction during the conversion of small numbers to scientific notation compared to converting very large numbers to scientific notation. For example, 500 requires the decimal point to move two places to the *left* to produce the scientific notation equivalent of 5×10^2 while 0.05 requires the decimal point to move two places to the *right* to produce 5×10^{-2}.

Other examples of numbers less than 1 converted to scientific notation are shown below:

$0.2 = 2 \times 0.1 = 2 \times 10^{-1}$
$0.25 = 2.5 \times 0.1 = 2.5 \times 10^{-1}$
$0.025 = 2.5 \times 0.01 = 2.5 \times 10^{-2}$
$0.002\,53 = 2.53 \times 0.001 = 2.53 \times 10^{-3}$

To convert the scientific notation of a number less than 1 back into a decimal value, the decimal point is moved to the *left* the same number of spaces as the superscript power, placing zeros as needed between the integer of the decimal fraction and the decimal point. For example, to convert 5.75×10^{-4} back to its decimal form, the decimal point is moved four spaces to the *left* and zeros are placed as needed in any spaces ("0.000 575").

2.6 Tips for Adding and Subtracting Decimal Numbers

Although calculators are readily available everywhere, there are still occasions when adding or subtracting decimal numbers by hand might be required. Because we have become so accustomed to doing all math on calculators, the ability to perform these operations by hand often results in inaccurate answers – much to the detriment of the patient. Even though properly entered data into a calculator reduces human error in performing decimal calculations, being able to perform these basic decimal operations accurately by hand is important for a well-educated and well-prepared veterinary technician. The following tips help reduce errors when doing decimal calculations by hand.

When writing out decimal numbers for adding or subtracting by hand, errors can be eliminated by doing three things:

1) put the numbers in columns for adding;
2) line up the numbers by putting the decimal points in a vertical line; and
3) use zeros as "placeholders" to help you visually make sure the columns are aligned.

For example, adding 12.3 + 0.01 + 1.075 can be confusing if the decimals are not lined up vertically and would likely result in an incorrect answer:

```
  12.3
   0.01
+  1.075
_____
```

Lining up the decimal points helps, but visually still looks a little odd:

12.3

0.01

+ 1.075

The use of trailing zeros as "placeholders" to the right of the decimal number makes it easier for the eye to track down the columns correctly and to add the appropriate numbers in each column:

12.300

0.010

+ 1.075

Remember that adding trailing zeros to the far right side of the decimal number (as long as it is to the *right* of the decimal point itself) doesn't change the value of the number.

Even though trailing zeros were used to set up the problem, trailing zeros should be eliminated from the actual answer. Although lining up the decimal points in a column and adding zeros as placeholders is *useful* for doing addition problems by hand, such alignment is *critical* to accurate subtract decimal numbers by hand. For example, 12.35 – 1.255 *looks* odd with the decimals lined up vertically if no zero placeholders are used. It seems even odder when you try to subtract the "five thousandths" from a blank space!

12.35

– 1.255

Putting the zero in as a placeholder makes the subtraction problem more familiar (borrow a "one" from the hundredths column and make the zero in the thousandths column a "ten"):

12.350

– 1.255

11.095

Remember that you can always check your subtraction answer by *adding* the answer (11.095) to the number above it (1.255) to determine if you arrive at the top number (12.350).

2.7 Tips for Multiplying Decimal Numbers

Unlike the necessity for lining up the columns of numbers discussed in addition and subtraction, multiplication of decimal numbers doesn't require vertical alignment. Instead, there are some simple rules for proper placement of the decimal point in the multiplication answer (the "product").

The method is fairly simple. Multiply the two numbers together as if the decimal points were not there (i.e. like a "whole number" multiplication problem). Then, count the *number* of digits (not their value) that are to the *right* of the decimal point in all numbers used in the problem, and move the decimal point of the answer that many places to the *left*. For example, if 2.3 × 4.55 were multiplied together, there are a total of three digits to the *right* of the decimal point. When the answer (the product) is calculated, the decimal point is then placed, or moved, three spaces to the left. For the example of 2.3 × 4.55, the problem is solved as shown below.

$$
\begin{array}{r}
2.3 \\
\times\, 4.55 \\
\hline
10.465
\end{array}
$$

Note that by moving the decimal point in the answer to the correct location by this method, we don't need to align the decimal points vertically in the multiplication problem when we set it up.

The same rules stated above for writing decimal numbers in general applies to the decimal products of decimal multiplication. If the product is a number less than 1, you need to add a zero in the "ones" place to emphasize the existence of the decimal point (".902" is written as "0.902"):

$$
\begin{array}{r}
90.2 \\
\times\, 0.01 \\
\hline
0.902
\end{array}
$$

What happens when a decimal multiplication gives a product (the answer) with only three digits but there are more than three digits to the right of the decimal point in the problem itself? For example, the multiplication problem of "0.25 × 0.15" will have a total of four digits located to the right of the decimal point. But the raw answer, before placement of the decimal point, comes out to "375," which only has three digits.

$$
\begin{array}{r}
0.25 \\
\times\, 0.15 \\
\hline
375
\end{array}
$$

In these situations, zeros are added to the *left* (not to the right) of the number until sufficient digits (four are needed for this case) have been added to allow proper placement of the decimal point. Because four digits are needed to properly place the decimal point for the answer to 0.25 × 0.15, an additional zero is placed to the *left* of the product, 375, giving "0375" in the raw form. The decimal point is then appropriately moved four places to the left to give the correct final answer.

$$
\begin{array}{r}
0.25 \\
\times\, 0.15 \\
\hline
0.0375
\end{array}
$$

As emphasized previously, a zero should be put in the ones column in this answer to call attention to the decimal point even though there is already a zero in the 1/10 column.

2.8 Tips for Dividing Decimal Numbers

Of all of the decimal calculations by hand, division problems often create the most errors. Practicing division by hand also increases a better understanding for what the correct answer should "look like" when doing division problems using a calculator. Thus, the veterinary technician should practice doing division problems by hand just to keep their dosage calculation skills sharp overall.

Three terms are often used to describe division problems: the dividend (the number being divided into parts), the divisor (the number telling how many parts there will be), and the quotient (the answer that tells how many pieces of the dividend are in each part). These are represented in long division bracket and the linear format of the division questions as shown below:

$$\text{divisor} \overline{)\text{dividend}}^{\text{quotient}} \qquad 5\overline{)10}^{\,2}$$

$$\text{dividend} \div \text{divisor} = \text{quotient} \qquad 10 \div 5 = 2$$

Remember that fractions are also considered to represent division problems – where the top part of the fraction would be the "dividend," the bottom part of the fraction would be the "divisor," and the result of dividing the top number by the bottom number would be the "quotient."

$$\frac{\text{dividend}}{\text{divisor}} = \text{quotient}$$

$$\frac{10}{5} = 2$$

Instead of using the terms associated with division problems, the components of the fraction are called the numerator (for the top) and the denominator (for the bottom). Manipulation of fraction problems will be discussed in greater detail in Chapter 3.

Decimal division is the same as whole integer division but with extra attention paid to the placement of the decimal point. In long division (using the division bracket) a decimal number in the divisor (the number outside the bracket "dividing" the dividend inside the bracket) requires moving the decimal point to the *right* both in the divisor *and* in the dividend located within the bracket even if the dividend is not a decimal number.

For example, the equation "82.5 ÷ 2.5 =" put into the division bracket would look like this:

$$2.5\overline{)82.5}^{\,?}$$

Because the divisor (the number outside the bracket) is a decimal fraction with a number in the tenths place, the divisor's decimal point and the dividend's decimal point are both moved one place to the right to make the divisor a whole number:

$$25.\overline{)825.}^{\,?}$$

The division problem is now solved in the same way as with any long division problem, making sure to place the decimal point in the quotient (the answer) directly above the position of the decimal in the dividend.

$$25.\overline{)825.}^{\,33.}$$

When dividing a number with decimal point, remember that the decimal point in the dividend inside the bracket is always moved in the same way as the divisor, regardless of the starting position of the decimal point in the dividend. If dividing $1.875 \div 0.15$, the decimal point is moved two places to the right to make the divisor a whole number and likewise the decimal point in the dividend is also moved the same number of positions:

$$0.15\overline{)1.875} \quad \text{becomes} \quad 15.\overline{)187.5} \quad \text{which solves to} \quad 15.\overline{)187.5}^{\,12.5}$$

Zeroes may have to be added to the dividend inside the bracket as placeholders when the decimal point is moved or as needed to perform the long division problem. Examples are shown below.

$$2 \div 15.34 \text{ becomes } 15.34\overline{)2} \text{ becomes } 1534.\overline{)2} \text{ becomes solves to } 15.34\overline{)200.00}^{\,0.13}$$

$$0.25 \div 25.115 \text{ becomes } 25.115\overline{)0.25} \text{ becomes } 25115.\overline{)250} \text{ which solves to } 25115.\overline{)250.00}^{\,0.001}$$

Note that sometimes the answer to a division problem terminates in a repeated number or in a series of numbers. For example, $100 \div 3 = 33.333\,333$ ... with the 3 s continuing onto infinity. Instead of rounding the number to $3.333\,33$ and stopping the trail of 3's at some arbitrary point (see "rounding" in Section 2.9), a repeating number or set of numbers in an answer can be indicated by placing a horizontal line above the number(s). The examples below illustrate this use:

$$1.3333333 = 1.3\overline{3}$$

$$1.272727 = 1.27\overline{27}$$

$$6.345345345 = 6.345\overline{345}$$

Veterinary technicians should be familiar enough with decimal operations to be able to predict a general answer in terms of the expected placement of the decimal point in the answer. For example, when the dividend number is divided by a divisor number that is greater than 1, the resulting answer quotient should always be smaller than the dividend. 10 divided by 5 yields 2; 2 is smaller in value than the original 10. However, when a dividend number is divided by a number less than 1 (0.5, 0.02, etc.) then the resulting quotient answer should be greater than the original dividend. 10 divided by 0.5 yields 20. As odd as this may seem, this equation is saying, how many pieces will result if each of the 10 pieces is split into half. By picturing 10 tablets being cut into half, we see intuitively that this would result in 20 half tablet pieces or twice as many pieces than what we started with. Visualizing mathematical operations into tangible materials that are multiplied or divided helps to conceptualize into concrete objects what is otherwise an abstract mathematical concept.

2.9 Accurately Rounding Decimal Numbers

Often the answers to division and multiplication problems are very long decimal numbers. For example, the equation "8 ÷ 1.23" yields an answer of 6.504 065. If this answer were the number of milliliters to be injected into an animal, it would be impractical to attempt to determine where the mark for 6.504 065 mL would be on the syringe. It then becomes necessary to accurately round the number to the nearest tenths or hundredths, etc.

To round a decimal number, identify the digit to the *right* of the place to which the number is to be rounded. For example, if a number is to be rounded to the nearest tenths place, the digit in the hundredths would be identified, or for a number rounded to the nearest hundredths place, the digit in the thousandths place would be identified, and so on.

If the identified integer in the adjacent place is 5 or greater, round the adjacent number (the slot to which the number is to be rounded – such as to the nearest 1/10th or nearest 1/100th) up by one unit. Thus, 1.85 rounded to the nearest 1/10th would be 1.9 because the integer in the 1/100ths place is 5 or greater requiring the addition of 1 to the 1/10th place. For 45.318 rounded to the nearest 1/100th, the presence of a number 5 or greater in the 1/1000ths place (the number in that position is 8 in this example) adds one to the 1/100ths place, producing the number 45.32. When rounding, any digits to the right of the place to which the number is rounded are *truncated* (dropped off) when the number is rounded. So 3.892 315 2 rounded to the nearest tenth is 3.9 and 7.869 237 23 rounded to the nearest 1/100th is 7.87. Remember that when the value of the number in the column to be rounded is increased by 1, the resulting number must numerically reflect that increase. Thus, 5.96 rounded to the nearest 1/10th would be 6.0 and 4.298 rounded to the nearest 1/100th would be 4.30 because of the addition of 1 to the rounded columns.

If the identified integer in the column to the right of the rounded column is less than 5, the number in the rounded column remains the same (it does *not* decrease). Thus 3.82 rounded to the nearest 1/10th is 3.8 and 6.722 rounded to the nearest 1/100th would be 6.72. Remember that the column to which the number is to be rounded must always contain an integer even if the integer is a trailing zero. Thus, 8.03 rounded to the nearest 1/10th is 8.0 and 9.004 rounded to the nearest 1/100th would be 9.00.

The same procedure is applied regardless of the place to which a number is being rounded. In the example below, 6.537 49 is rounded to the nearest whole number, the nearest tenth, the nearest hundredth, and the nearest thousandth. Check yourself to see if you agree with each rounding:

Whole number	6.537 49 = 7	Digit in the tenths place is 5 or greater
Nearest tenth	6.537 49 = 6.5	Digit in the hundredths place is less than 5
Nearest hundredth	6.537 49 = 6.54	Digit in the thousandths place is 5 or greater
Nearest thousandth	6.537 49 = 6.537	Digit in the ten-thousandths place is less than 5

2.10   Chapter 2 Practice Problems

1   What digit is in the thousandths location in the number 34 623.897 1?

2   Write the following numbers:

   A) "twenty-five and sixty-nine hundredths"
   B) "thirty-three thousand, four hundred fifty-two and six hundred and forty-eight thousandths"
   C) "three six seven point two one zero four"
   D) "twenty-six thousandths"

3   The veterinarian tells you to record the dose as "point zero one two grams." How do you write it?

4   Write the numerical value (e.g. 35.09 lb) described in each statement:

   A) "I need twelve point three zero cubic centimeters given to this dog." _____ cc
   B) "Put twenty-five one hundredths of a gram into the IV solution." _____ g
   C) "We removed one hundred thirty-two and three-tenths milliliters of fluid from his abdomen over the last 12 hours." _____ mL
   D) "The drug concentration was three thousandths of mg per milliliter." _____ mg/mL

5   What is wrong with the way each of the following numbers are written or spoken?

   A) 342.00
   B) .653
   C) The number 7.038 pronounced as "seven point three eight."
   D) The number 3.25 pronounced as "three and two tenths and five hundredths."

6   For each of the following, indicate which number is larger:

   A) 0.042 2 or 0.1936
   B) 0.005 21 or 0.000 212
   C) 0.499 or 0.5
   D) 0.0009 or 0.000 12
   E) 0.004 52 or 0.008

7   The drug's blood concentration is 0.0033 mcg of drug per milliliter of blood (mcg/mL). Is this concentration within the acceptable range of 0.02 and 0.04 mcg/mL?

8   The intravenous drip rate for the medication being administered to a patient indicates that the patient will receive 0.012 mg of drug per hour (mg/h). The patient needs between 0.0075 and 0.02 mg/h. Is this an acceptable drip rate for this drug?

9   Write the following numbers in scientific notation:

   A) 3673
   B) 235 233
   C) 5
   D) 86.6
   E) 5263.03

F) 0.7

G) 0.025

H) 0.000 430 4

I) 0.0200

J) 0.000 007 500

Note: for extra practice format all the answers in questions 11 through 19 in scientific notation.

10 Write the following in their decimal number format:

A) 2.4×10^2

B) 1.667×10^4

C) 5.3901×10^5

D) 1.003×10^1

E) $6.260\,045 \times 10^3$

F) 8.32×10^{-2}

G) 1.005×10^{-5}

H) $9.012\,403 \times 10^{-6}$

11 Calculate the answers for the following decimal problems, without a calculator:

A) $2.3 + 4.5 =$

B) $13.56 + 4.32 =$

C) $145.6 + 4.675 =$

D) $0.23 + 1.034 =$

E) $45.210 + 0.002\,476 =$

F) $54.3 - 44.7 =$

G) $362.65 - 4.29 =$

H) $3.5 - 2.1567 =$

I) $0.952 - 0.7 =$

J) $12.133 - 0.09\,875 =$

12 Calculate the total amounts (add or subtract) in each of the following statements:

A) "Adding 12.4 cc and 3.5 cc to the IV fluids increases the fluid by what volume?" _____ cc

B) "Removing 0.5 mL from the 33.5 mL solution leaves how many mL of fluid?" _____ mL

C) "Combining 4.5, 3.2, and 0.025 g of powders produces total of how many grams?" _____ g

D) "Taking out 3.5 tablets from the 55 you've dispensed leaves how many tablets?" _____ tablets

13 Calculate the answers for the following decimal problems, without a calculator:

A) $10.35 + 0.03 + 2.005 + 13.025 =$

B) $82.452 - 32.0031 =$

C) $0.003 + 0.100 + 1.0214 + 0.0901 =$

D) $0.03 - 0.000\,87 =$

E) $19.0003 + 0.031\,001 + 2.837\,99 + 0.006\,79 =$

14 Calculate the answers for the following decimal problems, without a calculator:

A) $2.0 \times 4.5 =$

B) $1.3 \times 5.0 =$

C) 23.4 × 4.15 =
D) 35.167 × 3.12 =
E) 40.02 × 18.15 =
F) 5.002 × 34.101 =
G) 0.9 × 8.2 =
H) 0.123 × 10.02 =
I) 3.1002 × 0.03 =
J) 34.620 × 0.023 =
K) 3.12 × 0.01 =
L) 52.002 × 3.002 =
M) 96.01 × 38.909 =
N) 57.219 × 0.009 =
O) 86.030 × 1.029 200 =
P) 166.003 × 0.003 99 =
Q) 0.0098 × 3.925 01 =
R) 366.900 × 3.009 =
S) 352.88 × 0.0097 =
T) 0.010 × 0.003 92 =

15 Calculate the answers for the following decimal problems, without a calculator:

A) 5$\overline{)10.5}$
B) 8$\overline{)0.125}$
C) 0.3$\overline{)3.69}$
D) 1.02$\overline{)2.048}$
E) 0.8042$\overline{)3.01088}$
F) 33.0$\overline{)200.05}$

16 Calculate the answers for the following decimal problems, without a calculator:

A) 55.5 ÷ 5.0 =
B) 7.0 ÷ 0.2 =
C) 72.0 ÷ 1.002 =
D) 19 001 ÷ 32.021 =
E) 0.002 ÷ 0.0003 =
F) 15.0020 ÷ 2.0202 =
G) 9.020 999 ÷ 3.0299 =
H) 0.0251 ÷ 0.0915 =
I) 0.0528 ÷ 5.300 05 =
J) 5.300 05 ÷ 0.0528 =

17 Answer the following questions by estimation only, without doing any calculations:

A) If 44 ÷ 2 = 22, then will 44 ÷ 0.2 equal 2.2 or 220?
B) If 616 ÷ 40 = 15.4, then will 616 ÷ 0.4 equal 1540 or 0.154?
C) If 0.024 ÷ 0.02 = 1.2, then will 0.024 ÷ 0.002 equal 12 or 0.12?

18 Round the following numbers to the place indicated:

A) 32.092 to nearest tenth
B) 1.174 39 to nearest hundredth

C) 8.500 2 to nearest whole number

D) 4259.999 to nearest thousand

E) 41.009 95 to nearest tenth

F) 819.273 to nearest hundred

G) 0.328 97 to nearest hundredth

H) 9.939 87 to nearest hundredth

I) 0.000 702 3 to nearest thousandth

J) 0.009 283 to nearest ten thousandth

K) 0.014 263 863 to nearest millionth

L) 2.192 837 55 to nearest hundred thousandth

M) 5.555 555 to nearest thousandth

19 Calculate the following answers, rounding to the place indicated, without a calculator:

A) $0.175 \div 2.3 =$ _____ , round to the nearest hundredth

B) $0.3 \times 6.732 =$ _____ , round to the nearest hundredth

3

Review of Key Math Fundamentals

Fractions

Fractions are used in many medical situations. For example, veterinarians may decide that they want to "reduce the flow rate of IV medication by half" or it may be necessary to "divide the dose into thirds" for safe administration to the patient. Even with the use of a calculator, the veterinary professional must still be able to understand the concept of fractions, how they are calculated, and how to transition between fraction numbers and decimal numbers.

3.1 Fundamentals of Working with Medical Math Fractions

The arrangement of a fraction simply communicates that a whole of "something" is going to be divided into smaller components. The bottom number in a fraction is the *denominator* and states into how many parts the whole is to be divided (1/2 means divided into two parts, 3/4 means divided into four parts, etc.). Figure 3.1 shows how two half (1/2) tablets represent two parts of a whole and when added together will produce one whole tablet. The top number in the fraction is the *numerator* and states how many of those parts or pieces there are to begin with (3/4 means there are three pieces, 2/5 means there are two, etc.). To keep the terms straight, remember that "denominator" begins with a "d" like in the word "down," and therefore the denominator is "down below the numerator."

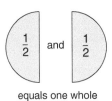

equals one whole

Figure 3.1 The denominator says into how many parts the whole is divided and the numerator tells how many of the individual parts there are. 1 tablet split into 2 pieces = two ½ pieces

Fractions not only represent the outcome of the division of a whole into parts, but they also constitute a mathematical operation. The fraction says, "divide the numerator by the denominator to produce a decimal number." Thus, the representation of "2/8" means "divide 2 by 8." In so doing 2/8 fraction becomes the decimal number 0.25. The conversion between decimals and fractions will be discussed later in this chapter.

Medical Mathematics and Dosage Calculations for Veterinary Technicians, Third Edition. Robert Bill.
© 2019 John Wiley & Sons, Inc. Published 2019 by John Wiley & Sons, Inc.
Companion website: www.wiley.com/go/bill/calculations

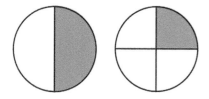

Figure 3.2 One half (1/2) of a tablet is a larger piece than one fourth (1/4) of the whole tablet

Remembering how changes in the fraction affect the value of the fraction allows the veterinary technician to estimate the general answer to calculations involving fractional division problems. Mathematically, *when the denominator increases, the value of the fraction decreases.* If a tablet were divided into halves and another tablet divided into fourths, the individual pieces of the tablet divided into fourths would be smaller than the individual pieces of the tablet divided into halves (see Figure 3.2). One piece of the four-way divided tablet is smaller than one piece of the two-way divided tablet, and therefore 1/4 has a smaller value than 1/2. If 1/4 is converted into a decimal number by dividing the numerator (top) by the denominator (bottom) the value of 0.25 is seen to be smaller than the value of 0.50, which is the value derived from dividing one by two in the fraction 1/2. Thus, 1/100th of a gram is far smaller than 1/10th of a gram, and 1/3rd of a mL is a far larger volume than 1/10th of a mL.

3.2 Working with Improper Fractions, Proper Fractions, and Mixed Numbers

A veterinary technician needs to give a half tablet to three different patients in the hospital. She removes a whole tablet and a previously sectioned half tablet from the bottle of tablets of the drug needed. She splits the whole into half and therefore now has three, half tablets to give to her patients. The number of tablets the technician has could be described as "three halves" and expressed as "3/2." Because the numerator (top number) is larger than the denominator, the "3/2" fraction is referred to as an *improper fraction*.

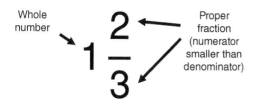

Figure 3.3 Anatomy of a mixed number: a whole number plus a proper fraction

Table 3.1 Examples of improper fractions converted to mixed numbers

Improper fraction	Mixed number
$\dfrac{6}{4}$	$1\dfrac{2}{4}$
$\dfrac{16}{5}$	$3\dfrac{1}{5}$
$\dfrac{32}{24}$	$1\dfrac{8}{24}$
$\dfrac{12}{9}$	$1\dfrac{3}{9}$
$\dfrac{64}{15}$	$4\dfrac{4}{15}$

Although mathematically accurate, improper fractions are not typically written in drug orders or medical records. Instead, the improper fraction is converted to a *mixed number*. A mixed number contains a whole number plus a *proper fraction* (a fraction where the numerator is *smaller* than the denominator). An example is shown in Figure 3.3.

To convert from an improper fraction to a mixed number, the numerator (top) is divided by the denominator (bottom) to obtain the whole number. The "leftover" from the division process becomes the proper fraction. For example, the improper fraction 5/3 would be changed by first dividing 5 by 3. We see that 3 goes into 5 only one time, so the whole number in the mixed number answer is going to be 1. When 3 goes into 5, there is are 2 left over; therefore, the fraction of the mixed number is going to be 2/3. The final answer is 1 and 2/3 (which can also be shown as $1\frac{2}{3}$). Other conversions of improper fractions are shown in Table 3.1. For safety reasons, when writing mixed numbers it is important that the whole number part is written so that the size of the written digits are significantly larger than those written in the fraction part. This will ensure that the mixed number fraction $1\frac{2}{3}$ is not mistaken for the improper fraction $\frac{12}{3}$.

It is important to remember that any number over 1 in a fraction is equivalent to that number. In other words, 4/1 as an improper fraction is equivalent to the whole number 4, 32/1 is equivalent to 32, and 128/1 is equal to 128. This concept will be important in discussing reciprocals later in this chapter.

If the conversion of the improper fraction to a mixed number results in no left over number after the division, then the value is represented only by the whole number. For example, 6/3 would have the value of 2 and 24/8 would have the value of 3.

If it is necessary to convert from a mixed number back into an improper fraction, the conversion process is reversed by multiplying instead of dividing. To convert the mixed number 2 and 1/3 back into an improper fraction, the denominator (bottom number) is multiplied by the whole number, then the numerator (top number) is added to give the total of the fractional parts. For the mixed number 2 and 1/3, the fraction's denominator 3 would be multiplied by the whole number 2 to get value 6 representing six fractional pieces. The 6 would be added to the numerator 1 in the fraction 1/3 to get 7, representing a total of seven fractional pieces. Thus, the improper fraction to represent 2 and 1/3 would be 7/3.

3.3 Equivalent Fractions in Medical Math

If a veterinary technician needed to give a half tablet of medication to a dog, but had to use tablets that had already been cut into quarters, he could put two of the quarter pieces together to form one half of a tablet, as shown in Figure 3.4.

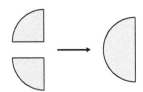

Figure 3.4 Two smaller quarter pieces put together equal one half piece

As shown in Figure 3.4, two fourths are equivalent to one half. This means that that a value of the fraction 2/4 is equivalent to the value of 1/2. Indeed, if 2 is divided by 4 and 1 is divided by 2 to produce the decimal equivalents for these two fractions, the value for both is 0.5. Thus one-half and two-fourths are said to be *equivalent fractions* because they numerically represent the same amount.

Identifying equivalent fractions sometimes is required when drug formulations are fractionated but the fraction is different than the fraction called for in the dose or the drug order (as in the example above). If you are given a fraction and you are required to determine equivalent fractions, it is simply a matter of multiplication and following the rule that "Whatever you do to the numerator, you must do to the denominator." In other words, to determine the equivalent fraction for 1/2 in fourths, the denominator (bottom part) would need to be multiplied by 2 to get 4 for the fourths. And because whatever is done to the denominator must be done to the numerator, the top is also multiplied by 2:

$$\frac{1}{2} \times \frac{2}{2} = \frac{1 \times 2}{2 \times 2} = \frac{2}{4}$$

Because any fraction where the numerator is the same as the denominator equals the value of 1 (2/2 = 1, 100/100 = 1, etc.) and because any number multiplied by 1 equals itself (5 × 1 = 5, 10 × 1 = 10, etc.), multiplying the fraction 1/2 by the fraction 2/2 (which has a value of 1) did not change the *value* of the fraction when it became 2/4. Thus 1/2 and 2/4 are equivalent fractions because they have the same value. If the fraction 1/2 was multiplied by 3/3, 4/4, 10/10, or 2000/2000, all your answers would have the same value as 1/2:

$$\frac{1}{2} \times \frac{3}{3} = \frac{1 \times 3}{2 \times 3} = \frac{3}{6}$$

$$\frac{1}{2} \times \frac{4}{4} = \frac{1 \times 4}{2 \times 4} = \frac{4}{8}$$

$$\frac{1}{2} \times \frac{10}{10} = \frac{1 \times 10}{2 \times 10} = \frac{10}{20}$$

$$\frac{1}{2} \times \frac{2000}{2000} = \frac{1 \times 2000}{2 \times 2000} = \frac{2000}{4000}$$

Therefore

$$\frac{1}{2} = \frac{3}{6} = \frac{4}{8} = \frac{10}{20} = \frac{2000}{4000}$$

3.4 Simplifying or Reducing Fractions

Fractions such as 2000/4000 are rather difficult to work with and are prone to errors when put into a calculator simply because the more digits there are to put into the calculator, the greater the likelihood of inaccurately entering the data. Also, it is difficult to translate a complex fraction like this into something practical such as a tablet fraction. How would a veterinary technician dispense 2000/4000 of a tablet? Certainly it would not require dividing a tablet into 4000 pieces and then counting out 2000 of them! Therefore, it is preferable to always use the simplest equivalent fraction in medical math.

To simplify or "reduce" fractions to a simpler equivalent fraction, the numerator and denominator are both divided by the same number remembering the "Whatever you do to the numerator, you must do to the denominator" rule. When numerators and denominators are divided, the resulting conversion must give whole numbers in both the numerator and denominator. Any whole number that can evenly be divided into *both* the numerator and denominator of the fraction is said to be a *common factor* for both numerator and denominator. The largest whole number that can be evenly divided into both numerator and denominator is the *greatest common factor*. The greatest common factor is sometimes also referred to in other calculation references as the greatest common divisor or the highest common factor.

For example, to simplify a fraction like 8/16, it's easy to see that 2, 4, and 8 can all be evenly divided into both the top and bottom numbers of the fraction with no remainders or leftovers. 2, 4, and 8 would be common factors and 8 would be the greatest common factor. Dividing the original fraction 8/16 by any of these common factors would result in a simpler or reduced fraction with an equivalent value of the original fraction.

$$\frac{8}{16} \div \frac{2}{2} = \frac{8 \div 2}{16 \div 2} = \frac{4}{8}$$

$$\frac{8}{16} \div \frac{4}{4} = \frac{8 \div 4}{16 \div 4} = \frac{2}{4}$$

$$\frac{8}{16} \div \frac{8}{8} = \frac{8 \div 8}{16 \div 8} = \frac{1}{2}$$

It may be difficult to immediately determine how fractions with large numbers can be simplified. However, first determine if both the numerator and the denominator are evenly divisible by some simple prime numbers (2, 3, or 5) and do an initial simplification. For example, the fraction 256/1024 seems daunting to simplify. But because the top and bottom numbers are both even, they can be divided by 2 to start the process of simplification.

$$\frac{256}{1024} \div \frac{2}{2} = \frac{256 \div 2}{1024 \div 2} = \frac{128}{512}$$

Repeat this process until the fraction is reduced to the simplest, but equivalent, form.

$$\frac{128}{512} \div \frac{2}{2} = \frac{64}{256}$$

$$\frac{64}{256} \div \frac{2}{2} = \frac{32}{128}$$

$$\frac{32}{128} \div \frac{2}{2} = \frac{16}{64}$$

$$\frac{16}{64} \div \frac{8}{8} = \frac{2}{8}$$

$$\frac{2}{8} \div \frac{2}{2} = \frac{1}{4}$$

Notice how as the numbers in the fraction got smaller it was easier to identify a larger common factor and to speed up the process of reducing the fraction.

Improper fractions (e.g. 24/16) can be simplified (or reduced) using the same steps outlined above or, as an alternative, the improper fraction can be converted to a mixed number before reducing just the fraction part of the mixed number. For example, the improper fraction 6/4 is equal to the mixed number 1 and 2/4. The 2/4 fraction is reduced to 1/2, producing the final answer of 1 and 1/2.

$$\frac{6}{4} = 1\frac{2}{4} = 1\frac{1}{2}$$

3.5 Adding Fractions in Medical Math

Adding fractions of tablets or medications is something veterinary professionals should be able to do accurately. It is not difficult to add together two fractions that have *common denominators*, in other words, where the lower digit in both fractions is the same. For fractions with common denominators, adding the two fractions together means simply adding *only* the numerators, keeping the common denominator the same. Picture having two 1/4 tablets on a tablet-counting tray. Pushing them together produces two quarters. The result of adding the fractions 1/4 + 1/4 would be the fraction 2/4, not 2/8. *Only* the numerator is added; the common denominator remains the *same*.

If, however, two fractions need to be added that do not have a common denominator, a conversion is required prior to adding. In some examples, one of the fractions in the addition problem needs to be converted to an equivalent fraction that results in both fractions in the problem having the same common denominator. In the example below, the 1/2 needs to be converted into the equivalent sixths because 1/6 cannot be converted into equivalent halves.

$$\frac{1}{2} + \frac{1}{6} = \frac{3}{6} + \frac{1}{6} = \frac{3+1}{6} = \frac{4}{6} \quad \text{which reduces to} \quad \frac{2}{3}$$

With some fractions the common denominator is not immediately obvious. For example, the addition of fractions 2/5 + 4/7 seems to require that both fractions be converted to equivalent fractions in order to find a common denominator. While producing a long list of equivalent fractions for both numbers and searching for a common denominator among the list could work, a much easier way to find a common denominator between the two fractions is to multiply the denominators from both fractions with each other and use the resulting product (answer) as the common denominator. The original individual fractions are then converted to equivalent fractions containing the common denominator and the fractions added together.

For the problem of 2/5 + 4/7, the common denominator would be found by multiplying 5 (from the 2/5 fraction) by 7 (from the 4/7 fraction) to give 35. 35 now becomes the common denominator for both fractions and they are changed to their equivalent fraction forms.

$$\frac{2}{5} + \frac{4}{7} = ??? \quad \text{use 35 as common denominator}$$

$$\frac{2}{5} \times \frac{7}{7} = \frac{14}{35} \quad \text{converts the } \frac{2}{5} \text{ fraction into common denominator fraction } \frac{14}{35}$$

$$\frac{4}{7} \times \frac{5}{5} = \frac{20}{35} \quad \text{converts the } \frac{4}{7} \text{ fraction into the common denominator fraction } \frac{20}{35}$$

$$\frac{14}{35} + \frac{20}{35} = \frac{14+20}{35} = \frac{34}{35}$$

Note that although the answer in this example cannot be reduced, as a general rule the answer fractions should be reduced if possible to a simpler form. Other examples of these types of calculations are shown in Table 3.2.

Mixed numbers with fractions can be added by either of two methods, one which converts the mixed number to improper fractions and then adds them, or the other which adds the whole numbers and the fractions separately. Either method is equally valid and is used according to one's preference.

Table 3.2 Examples of addition of fractions using common denominators

Original problem	Conversion of fraction #1	Conversion of fraction #2	Final problem form
$\frac{3}{7} + \frac{2}{4} = ???$	$\frac{3}{7} \times \frac{4}{4} = \frac{12}{28}$	$\frac{2}{4} \times \frac{7}{7} = \frac{14}{28}$	$\frac{12}{28} + \frac{14}{28} = \frac{26}{28} = \frac{13}{14}$
$\frac{6}{13} + \frac{5}{12} = ???$	$\frac{6}{13} \times \frac{12}{12} = \frac{72}{156}$	$\frac{5}{12} \times \frac{13}{13} = \frac{65}{156}$	$\frac{72}{156} + \frac{65}{156} = \frac{137}{156}$
$\frac{5}{9} + \frac{2}{5} = ???$	$\frac{5}{9} \times \frac{5}{5} = \frac{25}{45}$	$\frac{2}{5} \times \frac{9}{9} = \frac{18}{45}$	$\frac{25}{45} + \frac{18}{45} = \frac{43}{45}$

In the first method the mixed numbers are first converted into improper fractions, as described previously.

$$1\frac{1}{2} + 3\frac{3}{4} = ??? \quad \text{is converted to} \quad \frac{3}{2} + \frac{15}{4} = ???$$

Then a common denominator is identified and the addition operation performed as described previously.

$$\frac{3}{2} + \frac{15}{4} = ??? \quad \text{common denominator conversion to} \quad \frac{6}{4} + \frac{15}{4} = ???$$

$$\text{perform the addition operation}: \quad \frac{6}{4} + \frac{15}{4} = \frac{6+15}{4} = \frac{21}{4}$$

$$\text{convert the improper fraction back to mixed number}: \quad \frac{21}{4} = 5\frac{1}{4}$$

In the second method, a common denominator is identified for the fractions but the fractions are kept in their proper form within the mixed number.

$$1\frac{1}{2} + 3\frac{3}{4} = ??? \quad \text{fractions are converted to common denominator}, \text{giving } 1\frac{2}{4} + 3\frac{3}{4} = ???$$

The fractions themselves are then added together, and then, separately, the whole numbers are added together.

$$1\frac{2}{4} + 3\frac{3}{4} = ??? \quad \text{add whole numbers then add fractions}: 1 + 3 = 4 \text{ and } \frac{2}{4} + \frac{3}{4} = \frac{5}{4}$$

If the addition of the fractions results in an improper fraction, convert the improper fraction to a mixed number. Finally, add the mixed number to the sum of the whole numbers.

$$\frac{5}{4} \text{ is converted to mixed number } 1\frac{1}{4}$$

$$\text{add mixed number to total for whole numbers}: \quad 1\frac{1}{4} + 4 = 5\frac{1}{4}$$

3.6 Subtracting Fractions in Medical Math

As with fraction addition, fraction subtraction requires all fractions in the problem to have a common denominator. Finding the common denominator for the fractions in the problem is done using the same procedures described above for addition. For example, for the operation 2/3 minus 1/2, the common denominator for both fractions must be found, the fractions converted to fractions with the common denominator, and then the problem solved by subtracting *only* the numerators.

$$\frac{2}{3} - \frac{1}{2} = ???$$

convert fractions to common denominator : $\dfrac{2}{3} - \dfrac{1}{2} = \dfrac{4}{6} - \dfrac{3}{6}$

solve by subtracting numerators : $\dfrac{4}{6} - \dfrac{3}{6} = \dfrac{4-3}{6} = \dfrac{1}{6}$

In subtracting mixed numbers, the first technique described above for adding mixed numbers should be used to avoid unnecessary complexity when fractions need to "carry over" a value to accurately subtract fractions. By first converting the mixed numbers into improper fractions with the same common denominator, the operation goes more smoothly.

$$6\dfrac{1}{3} - 4\dfrac{1}{4} = ???$$

convert to improper fractions : $\dfrac{19}{3} - \dfrac{17}{4} = ???$

find common denominator and convert fractions to it : $\dfrac{19}{3} \times \dfrac{4}{4} = \dfrac{76}{12}$ and $\dfrac{17}{4} \times \dfrac{3}{3} = \dfrac{51}{12}$

then perform the subtraction operation : $\dfrac{76}{12} - \dfrac{51}{12} = \dfrac{76-51}{12} = \dfrac{25}{12}$

$\dfrac{25}{12}$ converts back to mixed number : $2\dfrac{1}{12}$

3.7 Multiplying Fractions in Medical Math

In some ways, the mechanics involved with fraction multiplication and division are easier than fraction addition or subtraction. To multiply two fractions, multiply the numerators together and use that number for the numerator of the answer, then multiply the denominators together and use that answer for the denominator of the answer. Some examples shown below:

$\dfrac{1}{2} \times \dfrac{2}{3} = \dfrac{1 \times 2}{2 \times 3} = \dfrac{2}{6}$ which simplifies to $\dfrac{1}{3}$

$\dfrac{3}{4} \times \dfrac{4}{5} = \dfrac{3 \times 4}{4 \times 5} = \dfrac{12}{20}$ which simplifies to $\dfrac{3}{5}$

$\dfrac{10}{16} \times \dfrac{2}{3} = \dfrac{10 \times 2}{16 \times 3} = \dfrac{20}{48}$ which simplifies to $\dfrac{5}{12}$

Improper fractions are multiplied together using the same procedure as proper fractions, described above, without having to change their form. As a general rule, if the answer is an improper fraction, it should be converted to a mixed number.

When multiplying a whole number by a fraction, the whole number can be converted to its equivalent valued fraction (e.g. 2 = 2/1, 15 = 15/1) and multiplied as other fractions previously described, or the whole number can simply be multiplied with the rest of the numerators (top numbers). The numbers used in the equations below are equivalent in value.

$$\frac{3}{1} \times \frac{2}{7} \quad \text{is the same as} \quad 3 \times \frac{2}{7} = \frac{6}{7}$$

If one or more mixed numbers are to be multiplied, it is easiest just to convert any mixed numbers to improper fractions, then multiply the improper fractions together as would be done with any fractions. Do not forget to convert the improper fraction answer back to a mixed number and reduce the fraction if needed. See the example below:

$$2\frac{1}{4} \times 3\frac{1}{2} = ???$$

convert mixed numbers to improper fractions :
$$2\frac{1}{4} \times 3\frac{1}{2} = \frac{9}{4} \times \frac{7}{2}$$

multiply :
$$\frac{9}{4} \times \frac{7}{2} = \frac{9 \times 7}{4 \times 2} = \frac{63}{8}$$

convert the improper fraction back to a mixed number :
$$\frac{63}{8} = 7\frac{7}{8}$$

When multiplying fractions together, especially if multiplying several fractions together at once, the numerators and the denominators can become very large, making the fractions difficult to work with and the answers hard to reduce or simplify. For example, multiplying $\frac{3}{8} \times \frac{4}{7} \times \frac{6}{10}$ produces the following large answer that has to be reduced:

$$\frac{3}{8} \times \frac{4}{7} \times \frac{6}{10} = \frac{72}{560}$$

The problem is easier to solve if the fractions can be simplified to equivalent fractions with smaller denominators *before* performing the multiplication.

Before discussion about how this process is performed, it is necessary to emphasize an important mathematical principle about multiplication: it does not matter in what order items are multiplied; the answer will be the same. Thus, all of the problems shown below produce the same answer:

$$10 \times 2 \times 4 = 80$$

$$4 \times 2 \times 10 = 80$$

$$2 \times 10 \times 4 = 80$$

Because multiplication of fractions involves multiplying all the numerators to get the numerator of the answer and then multiplying all of the denominators to get the answer's denominator, it does not really matter in what order the numerators or the denominators are multiplied. Thus, each of these fraction multiplication problems shown below produce the same answer:

$$\frac{3}{4} \times \frac{1}{2} \times \frac{5}{6} = \frac{15}{48}$$

$$\frac{1}{6} \times \frac{5}{4} \times \frac{3}{2} = \frac{15}{48}$$

$$\frac{5}{2} \times \frac{1}{4} \times \frac{3}{6} = \frac{15}{48}$$

This principle of being able to shift the order of the numbers multiplied allows for simplification of the fractions to be multiplied.

In the following problem, the numbers in the fractions being multiplied are rearranged to allow reducing or simplifying of the fractions in the calculation:

$$\frac{3}{10} \times \frac{2}{3} \times \frac{5}{6} = \frac{3 \times 2 \times 5}{10 \times 3 \times 6}$$

the numerators are rearranged to make reducible fractions : $\dfrac{5 \times 3 \times 2}{10 \times 3 \times 6}$

these fractions are then reduced to their lowest form : $\dfrac{5}{10} \times \dfrac{3}{3} \times \dfrac{2}{6} = \dfrac{1}{2} \times \dfrac{1}{1} \times \dfrac{1}{3}$

multiply to find the answer : $\dfrac{1}{2} \times \dfrac{1}{1} \times \dfrac{1}{3} = \dfrac{1}{6}$

If the original problem had been multiplied before reducing, the answer would have been 30/180, which is a much more cumbersome fraction to deal with. By taking a few seconds to simplify the fraction, the answer either does not have to be reduced after it has been multiplied, or if it must be reduced, it is far easier to do so.

It is not necessary to physically rearrange the numbers of the fractions to do this technique. Instead, numbers in the numerator that are factors of numbers in the denominator, and vice versa, can be visually identified and reduced before carrying out the multiplication problem.

$$\frac{3}{10} \times \frac{2}{3} \times \frac{5}{6} = ???$$

the 3 in the numerator cancels with the 3 in the denominator : $\dfrac{\mathbf{3}}{10} \times \dfrac{2}{\mathbf{3}} \times \dfrac{5}{6} = \dfrac{1}{10} \times \dfrac{2}{\mathbf{1}} \times \dfrac{5}{6}$

the 5 in the numerator reduces the 10 in the denominator : $\dfrac{1}{\mathbf{10}} \times \dfrac{2}{1} \times \dfrac{\mathbf{5}}{6} = \dfrac{1}{\mathbf{2}} \times \dfrac{2}{1} \times \dfrac{\mathbf{1}}{6}$

the 2 in the numerator reduces the 6 in the denominator : $\dfrac{1}{2} \times \dfrac{\mathbf{2}}{1} \times \dfrac{1}{\mathbf{6}} = \dfrac{1}{2} \times \dfrac{\mathbf{1}}{1} \times \dfrac{1}{\mathbf{3}}$

multiply the reduced, simplfied equation : $\dfrac{1}{2} \times \dfrac{1}{1} \times \dfrac{1}{3} = \dfrac{1}{6}$

The rule for reducing or simplifying fractions is the same rule stated previously: "Whatever you do to the numerator, you must do to the denominator." If a number among the numerator numbers is reduced in half, a number among the denominator numbers must also be reduced by half. As comfort is gained with practice multiplying fractions, this technique to simplify fractions before multiplying will become second nature.

3.8 Dividing Fractions in Medical Math

To simplify the concepts of division of fractions, the concept and mathematical rules pertaining to the *reciprocal* must be thoroughly understood. The *reciprocal of a fraction is the fraction flipped upside down.*

The reciprocal of $\frac{3}{5}$ is $\frac{5}{3}$

The reciprocal of $\frac{7}{8}$ is $\frac{8}{7}$

Rule 1 for reciprocals: Any fraction that is multiplied by its reciprocal equals 1.

$\frac{3}{5} \times \frac{5}{3} = \frac{15}{15}$ this reduces to $\frac{1}{1} = 1$

Rule 2 for reciprocals: The reciprocal of a whole number is 1 over that whole number and vice versa.

The reciprocal of 6 is $\frac{1}{6}$

The reciprocal of 372 is $\frac{1}{372}$

The reciprocal of $\frac{1}{18}$ is 18

Reciprocals play an essential role in fraction division because fraction division is actually multiplication of the reciprocal. This can be illustrated by imagining splitting a half tablet into two equal parts. The result of this split would be two quarter-sized pieces. Mathematically, the splitting of a half tablet in two to produce a quarter tablet would be represented as:

$\frac{1}{2} \div 2 = \frac{1}{4}$

It is counterintuitive to divide a number like 2 into smaller parts and result in a "larger" number of 4, until it is remembered that a larger denominator (bottom part of fraction) actually equates to a smaller value. So even though this is a division operation resulting in a smaller value, it appears that mathematically multiplying "2 × 2" was somehow used to create the 4 in the answer's denominator.

Indeed, fraction division actually involves multiplication using the *reciprocal* of the second number. In this case, the reciprocal of the second number 2 is 1/2.

$$\frac{1}{2} \div 2 \quad \text{means} \quad \frac{1}{2} \times \frac{1}{2} = \frac{1 \times 1}{2 \times 2} = \frac{1}{4}$$

Therefore, the key to dividing a fraction by a number is to convert the second number to its reciprocal and then to *multiply* the numbers together, following the rules for multiplication that were used in Section 3.7. A general formula that applies to dividing any fraction "*A/B*" by a whole number "*C*" is:

$$\frac{A}{B} \div C = \frac{A}{B} \times \frac{1}{C}$$

The same general rule applies to dividing whole numbers by fractions or fractions by fractions. Table 3.3 shows how fractional division problems are set up as fractional multiplication problems to be solved.

When dividing a mixed number by a fraction or when dividing a number by a mixed number, always convert the mixed number to an improper fraction first. Once the mixed numbers are converted to improper fractions, multiply the first number by the reciprocal of the second fraction as done previously. The resulting quotient (answer) should be simplified or reduced and converted back to a mixed number if necessary.

Notice that while canceling out the numerators with corresponding denominators was advocated for simplifying multiplication problems, it cannot be used in the same way to simplify fractional division *before* the original division problem is converted to its multiplication format. For example, in the fractional division 3/5 divided by 2/3 it appears to be able to simplify to 1/5 divided by 2/1. However, this results in the incorrect answer:

$$\frac{3}{5} \div \frac{2}{3} = ???$$

$$\frac{3}{5} \div \frac{2}{3} = \frac{1}{5} \div \frac{2}{1}$$

converts to multiplication problem $\frac{1}{5} \times \frac{1}{2} = \frac{1}{10}$ but gives an incorrect answer

Therefore, do *not* simplify division problems until after the problem has been converted to the multiplication format for solving.

Table 3.3 Fractional division is conducted by converting to fractional multiplication operations.

Original division problem	Multiplication format used to solve the problem
$\frac{2}{3} \div 8 =$	$\frac{2}{3} \times \frac{1}{8} = \frac{2}{24} = \frac{1}{12}$
$\frac{3}{5} \div \frac{2}{3} =$	$\frac{3}{5} \times \frac{3}{2} = \frac{9}{10}$
$16 \div \frac{4}{5} =$	$16 \times \frac{5}{4} = 4 \times \frac{5}{1} = 4 \times 5 = 20$

When a sequence of fractions are divided (for example, 2/5 divided by 1/2 divided by 1/4), the first number retains its form but all other subsequent fractions are reciprocated.

$$\frac{2}{5} \div \frac{1}{2} \div \frac{1}{4} \quad \text{is the same as} \quad \frac{2}{5} \times \frac{2}{1} \times \frac{4}{1}$$

$$\frac{2}{5} \times \frac{2}{1} \times \frac{4}{1} = \frac{2}{5} \times 2 \times 4 = \frac{16}{5} = 3\frac{1}{5}$$

When performing fractional math division on calculators, the reciprocal method can be performed as described above. Or, if the calculator has a group function, the first fraction's numerator can be divided by its denominator and then divided by the quotient *only* (not the individual parts) of the second fraction's division. For example, in using a calculator to divide 2/5 by 1/8 the following steps would be done:

1) divide 2 by 5, which gives 0.4 and save it
2) divide 1 by 8, which gives 0.125 and save it
3) divide 0.4 by 0.125 and get 3.2 for the answer

It would be easier to *multiply* the 2/5 by the reciprocal of 1/8 to get the answer.

1) 8 is the reciprocal of 1/8
2) $2 \times 8 = 16$ for the numerator of the answer
3) $5 \times 1 = 5$ for the denominator of the answer
4) final fraction answer is 16/5 which is 3.2

As a general rule, fractional division is far easier to perform as multiplication functions, especially for serial division problems which are commonly found in many dosage calculations.

3.9 Conversion Between Fractions and Decimals

Often conversion between fractions and decimals is required when calculating tablets or liquid volumes doses using a calculator. For example, the veterinarian might request that the drug dose for a patient with renal disease be decreased by one-third, which would need to be translated into decimal numbers to use a calculator to determine the adjusted dose. Another example would be when a dose is calculated on the calculator giving an answer as a decimal number that has to be converted to the nearest half or quarter tablet. Therefore, understanding how to quickly convert from a decimal number to a common fraction, and back, is a skill the veterinary technician should have.

Converting a fraction to decimal is much easier than doing the reverse operation. The simplest means to convert from a fraction to a decimal number is to divide the numerator by the denominator, as described in Section 3.1. For example, the fraction 1/4 is converted to the decimal number 0.25 by dividing the 1 in the numerator by the 4 in the denominator. The same would be true for 3/4, resulting in the decimal number 0.75. Some fraction to decimal conversions are used frequently in many aspects of veterinary medicine and it is an advantage for the veterinary technician to remember these particular conversions without having to calculate them. These conversions are shown in Table 3.4.

To convert mixed numbers to a decimal number, either the mixed number is first converted to an improper fraction or the fraction part of the mixed number is converted to its decimal equivalent and then added to the whole number. Both process are shown below.

Table 3.4 Common fraction to decimal conversions the technician should know.

Common fraction	Decimal number equivalent
$\frac{1}{2}$	0.5
$\frac{1}{4}$	0.25
$\frac{3}{4}$	0.75
$\frac{1}{3}$	0.333
$\frac{2}{3}$	0.667 (rounded)
$\frac{1}{5}$	0.2
$\frac{1}{8}$	0.125
$\frac{1}{10}$	0.1

$$1\frac{1}{4} \rightarrow \text{converted to improper fraction } \frac{5}{4} \rightarrow \text{converted to decimal by division} \rightarrow 1.25$$

or

$$1\frac{1}{4} \rightarrow \text{convert fraction } \frac{1}{4} \text{ only to decimal } 0.25 \rightarrow \text{added 0.25 to whole number } 1 \rightarrow 1.25$$

When a tablet dose is calculated using a calculator, the decimal answer must be translated into the number of tablets or fractions of tablets to be administered to the patient. For example, a student calculated a dose and found she had to give 0.75 of a tablet. How was the student going to determine how the tablet should be cut to give the appropriate dose?

To convert a decimal number to a fraction, start by writing it as a number over 10, 100, 1000, or whatever number corresponds to the right-most "decimal place" the number occupies. For example, the decimal number 0.75 corresponds to 75/100 because "75" occupies the hundredths place. Other examples are shown below.

$$0.7 = \frac{7}{10}$$

$$0.35 = \frac{35}{100}$$

$$0.493 = \frac{493}{1000}$$

$$0.8647 = \frac{8647}{10\,000}$$

The number is then reduced to its simplest form by dividing the numerator and the denominator by the same common factor number, as described in Section 3.4.

$$0.64 = \frac{64}{100} \text{ which reduces to } \frac{64 \div 2}{100 \div 2} = \frac{32}{50}$$

$$\frac{32 \div 2}{50 \div 2} = \frac{16}{25}$$

If a decimal number is greater than 1, it can be converted to a mixed number (a whole number and a fraction). The numbers to the *right* of the decimal point are converted to a fraction as described above, then added to the whole number comprised of the digits to the *left* of the decimal point to produce the mixed number. To convert the decimal number 3.25 to a fraction, the digits to the right of the decimal point are converted to a fraction:

$$0.25 = \frac{25}{100} = \frac{5}{20} = \frac{1}{4}$$

The fraction is then added to the whole number as represented by the digits to the left of the decimal point to produce the mixed number:

$$3.25 = 3 + 0.25 = 3 + \frac{1}{4} = 3\frac{1}{4}$$

As illustrated by this number above, no calculator would be needed for the decimal to fraction conversion if the technician memorized the basic fraction conversions in Table 3.4 and simply recognized that 0.25 is equivalent to the fraction 1/4.

3.10   Rounding Fractions in Medical Math

A veterinary technician determined the tablet dose for a dog to be 0.3125. When she converted the decimal number to the fraction it came out to 5/16 of a tablet. However, in practical terms, it would be very difficult to divide a tablet of medication into 5/16 of a tablet. Therefore, it is important to be able to accurately round fractions to the nearest half or quarter tablet.

The rounding is most easily done while the dose is still in the decimal number form. The decimal number answer is simply rounded to the nearest 0.5 or whole number, whichever is closer. Typically tablets are not broken into pieces smaller than halves; however, there are some occasions where human medications are being used on small dogs or cats where the tablet must be broken into quarters. In those situations the decimal number would need to be rounded to the nearest whole number, 0.25, 0.5, or 0.75 corresponding to a whole tablet, quarter tablet, half tablet, or three quarter tablet.

For example, the veterinary technician calculated a dose of drug for a dog to be 4.30 tablets per dose. The tablet is scored so that it can be easily divided into quarters, therefore the "0.30" component of the 4.30 would need to be rounded to the nearest quarter tablet (0.25, 0.50, 0.75, or 1.00). The 0.30 component of the decimal number is closest to 0.25; therefore, the 4.30 tablet dose is rounded "down" to 4.25. The 0.25 is equivalent to 1/4 therefore this animal is going to receive 4 and 1/4 tablets per dose.

If the dose calculation came out to 2.35 tablets and the tablets were only readily divided into halves and not quarters, the dose would have to be rounded to the nearest half or whole number. In this case, the decimal fraction of 0.35 is closer to 0.50 (there is a 0.15 difference) than it is to the whole tablet 0.00 (there is a 0.35 difference). Therefore, the 2.35 tablet dose is rounded "up" to 2.50. Because the veterinary technician recognizes that 2.50 is the same value as 2.5, and that the decimal fraction 0.5 is the same as the fraction 1/2, the technician correctly concluded that the appropriate dose was 2 and 1/2 tablets.

If presented with a fraction such as 5/16 that must be rounded to the nearest quarter or half, the fraction is first converted to its decimal equivalent. The decimal fraction is rounded to the nearest 0.25 or 0.50 increment as necessary, then converted back to the fraction form. For example, if the fraction 5/16 needs to be rounded to the nearest 1/4 tablet, it is first converted to its decimal form by dividing 5 by 16 to get 0.3125. The 0.3125 is closer to 0.2500 than it is to 0.5000 (verify this mathematically if needed). Therefore, 0.3125 would be rounded down to 0.25, converted back to the fraction of 25/100, and simplified to 1/4.

Note that dose rounding typically moves the dose up or down to the nearest fraction. A common misconception is that the rounding always goes down (or in some cases the rounding always goes up). With the exception of a few highly toxic drugs where rounding down is the prudent way to adjust the drug's dose, rounding of doses is always done to the nearest required fraction or whole.

3.11   Chapter 3 Practice Problems

1   True or false?

A) 1/3 is greater than 1/4
B) 1/10 is greater than 1/5
C) 1/16 is greater than 1/32
D) 2/3 is greater than 2/4
E) 3/10 is greater than 3/5
F) 10/16 is greater than 10/32

2   Write the equivalent fractions:

A) $\dfrac{1}{2} = \dfrac{???}{4} = \dfrac{???}{16} = \dfrac{???}{100}$

B) $\dfrac{1}{3} = \dfrac{???}{12} = \dfrac{???}{33} = \dfrac{???}{123}$

C) $\dfrac{2}{5} = \dfrac{???}{15} = \dfrac{???}{55} = \dfrac{???}{250}$

D) $\dfrac{7}{8} = \dfrac{???}{64} = \dfrac{???}{96} = \dfrac{???}{320}$

E) $2\dfrac{13}{16} = 2\dfrac{???}{64} = 2\dfrac{???}{480} = 2\dfrac{???}{3600}$

3   Reduce (simplify) the following fractions:

A) $\dfrac{4}{10}$

B) $\dfrac{6}{16}$

C) $\dfrac{24}{36}$

D) $\dfrac{36}{42}$

E) $\dfrac{72}{12}$

F) $\dfrac{73}{1}$

G) $2\dfrac{4}{8}$

H) $5\dfrac{24}{16}$

4   The following amounts were the results of dosage calculations. Simplify each fraction to its simplest form:

A) $\dfrac{8}{100}$ g

B) $\dfrac{45}{125}$ kg

C) $\dfrac{56}{128}$ kg

D) $\dfrac{512}{768}$ L

E) $\dfrac{19}{57}$ g

5   Solve the following fraction addition problems, expressing the answers in fractions:

A) $\dfrac{2}{8} + \dfrac{3}{8} =$

B) $\dfrac{3}{6} + \dfrac{6}{18} =$

C) $\dfrac{4}{48} + \dfrac{23}{24} =$

D) $\dfrac{3}{14} + \dfrac{35}{56} =$

E) $\dfrac{4}{12} + \dfrac{7}{36} =$

F) $\dfrac{32}{16} + \dfrac{14}{28} =$

G) $1\dfrac{3}{5} + \dfrac{49}{10} =$

H) $3\dfrac{14}{8} + 5\dfrac{24}{5} =$

I) $\dfrac{13}{8} + 4 + \dfrac{8}{24} =$

J) $1\dfrac{1}{2} + 3\dfrac{3}{4} + 12\dfrac{7}{8} + \dfrac{24}{36} =$

6   Solve the following fraction subtraction problems, expressing the answers in fractions:

A) $\dfrac{8}{16} - \dfrac{5}{16} =$

B) $\dfrac{4}{10} - \dfrac{7}{40} =$

C) $\dfrac{14}{28} - \dfrac{3}{14} =$

D) $\dfrac{43}{12} - \dfrac{31}{18} =$

E) $\dfrac{32}{64} - \dfrac{45}{128} =$

F) $2\dfrac{3}{6} - 1\dfrac{8}{24} =$

G) $8\dfrac{1}{4} - 5\dfrac{3}{4} =$

H) $12\dfrac{1}{2} - 9\dfrac{3}{4} =$

I) $\dfrac{38}{12} - 1\dfrac{14}{8} =$

J) $3\dfrac{12}{8} - 1\dfrac{2}{12} =$

7 Solve the following fraction multiplication problems, expressing the answers in fractions:

A) $\dfrac{1}{4} \times \dfrac{1}{2} =$

B) $\dfrac{3}{8} \times \dfrac{5}{6} =$

C) $\dfrac{32}{3} \times \dfrac{3}{5} =$

D) $\dfrac{2}{5} \times \dfrac{16}{10} =$

E) $\dfrac{14}{4} \times \dfrac{26}{12} =$

F) $5 \times \dfrac{5}{6} =$

G) $\dfrac{32}{18} \times 4 =$

H) $2\dfrac{2}{3} \times 4\dfrac{5}{6} =$

I) $1\dfrac{1}{2} \times 3\dfrac{3}{4} =$

J) $12\dfrac{1}{4} \times 24\dfrac{1}{2} \times 4\dfrac{3}{4} =$

8   Solve the following fraction division problems, expressing the answers in fractions:

A) $\dfrac{1}{2} \div \dfrac{3}{4} =$

B) $\dfrac{4}{5} \div \dfrac{1}{5} =$

C) $\dfrac{3}{8} \div 2 =$

D) $\dfrac{16}{32} \div \dfrac{2}{8} =$

E) $1\dfrac{1}{2} \div \dfrac{3}{8} =$

F) $3\dfrac{1}{4} \div 8 =$

G) $12\dfrac{3}{16} \div 2\dfrac{1}{8} =$

H) $39\dfrac{12}{32} \div 5\dfrac{14}{16} =$

I) $342\dfrac{12}{16} \div 23\dfrac{34}{64} =$

J) $\dfrac{125}{15} \div 7\dfrac{8}{50} =$

9   Convert the following fractions to decimal numbers:

A) $\dfrac{3}{4} =$

B) $\dfrac{9}{10} =$

C) $\dfrac{7}{8} =$

D) $\dfrac{23}{35} =$

E) $\dfrac{48}{16} =$

F) $\dfrac{39}{24} =$

G) $2\dfrac{3}{4} =$

H) $23\dfrac{13}{32} =$

I) $45\dfrac{15}{18} =$

J) $231\dfrac{81}{125} =$

10 Convert the following decimal numbers to the nearest quarter tablet. Write the answer as a proper quarter or half fraction, whole number, or mixed number.

A) 0.38 tablet = _____ tablet
B) 1.799 tablets = _____ tablets
C) 3.0921 tablets = _____ tablets
D) 12.645 tablets = _____ tablets
E) 5.81022 tablets = _____ tablets

11 Round each fraction to the nearest quarter tablet. Write the answer as a proper quarter or half fraction, whole number, or mixed number.

A) $\dfrac{7}{16} =$

B) $\dfrac{17}{64} =$

C) $\dfrac{23}{5} =$

D) $6\dfrac{2}{3} =$

E) $23\dfrac{17}{32} =$

12 Over the next several days, a dog is going to be on a decreasing dose of prednisolone tablets. The veterinarian has provided you with the daily doses below. The veterinarian is not going to dispense a fraction of tablet, so you need to determine how many *whole* tablets need to be dispensed to the owner to cover the dosage regimen listed.

A) Days 1–3: Give one and a half tablet twice daily
B) Days 4–6: Give one and a half tablet daily
C) Days 7–9: Give three-quarters of a tablet daily
D) Days 10–14: Give one-quarter of a tablet daily

13 The following written directions for an intravenously administered chemotherapy have been left for you by a very meticulous veterinarian. Determine how much of the drug in milligrams is needed for this patient.

"The regular dose is 36 mg. Because of his poorly functioning kidneys, give one-half of the regular dose. Add to that calculated dose three and three-quarters mg to compensate for the amount of drug that will stick to the intravenous infusion set. But remove 1.825 mg from this total calculated amount just to be safe."

4

Review of Key Math Fundamentals

Percentages

OBJECTIVES

The student will be able to:

1) accurately convert percentages to decimal numbers and vice versa,
2) accurately convert percentages to fractions and vice versa,
3) correctly interpret verbal and written orders involving percentages, and
4) correctly adjust doses using percentages.

Percentages are frequently used to describe how dosages are to be increased or decreased to meet the condition of a patient. It is important that the veterinary professional be able to understand percentages well enough to interpret drug orders, to use percentages to properly calculate changes in drug dosages, and to be able to accurately convert percentages to fractions or decimals.

4.1 Conversion of Percentages to Fractions

A percentage of a number is another way of saying that there are a certain number of items out of 100. In other words, if 5% of the tablets in a group of tablets are colored orange, the percentage number is saying that 5 tablets out of 100 are orange in color. Therefore, percentage (%) is another way of saying "out of 100" or "for every 100."

Because percentages represent "X out of 100," they can be represented as a fraction of "X" over "100." For example, 25% can be converted to an equivalent fraction form as follows:

$$25\% = \frac{25}{100} \text{ which can be simplified to}$$

$$\frac{25}{100} = \frac{5}{20} = \frac{1}{4}$$

Therefore, "25% of an administered dose of medication" would be equivalent to "1/4 of an administered dose of medication."

Medical Mathematics and Dosage Calculations for Veterinary Technicians, Third Edition. Robert Bill.
© 2019 John Wiley & Sons, Inc. Published 2019 by John Wiley & Sons, Inc.
Companion website: www.wiley.com/go/bill/calculations

If the percentage is represented as a decimal fraction (e.g. 5.25, 10.3), then the percentage is put into the fraction in the form of X over 100 and then the numerator and the denominator are multiplied by a value of 10, 100, or 1000, etc. to make the decimal numerator a whole number. Examples are shown below:

$$12.5\% = \frac{12.5}{100} \text{ which is then multiplied}: \frac{12.5}{100} \times \frac{10}{10} = \frac{125}{1000}$$

$$\text{and simplified}: \frac{25}{200} = \frac{5}{40} = \frac{1}{8}$$

$$6.25\% = \frac{6.25}{100} \text{ which is then multiplied}: \frac{6.25}{100} \times \frac{100}{100} = \frac{625}{10000}$$

$$\text{and simplified}: \frac{125}{2000} = \frac{25}{400} = \frac{5}{80} = \frac{1}{16}$$

Therefore, 12.5% of an amount is equivalent to 1/8 of the amount and 6.25% equals 1/16. The percentage equivalents for some commonly used fractions should be memorized to facilitate the efficiency of performing simple calculations. Common fractions and their percentage and decimal number equivalent are shown in Table 4.1.

4.2 Conversion Between Percentages and Decimal Numbers

Percentages are best used in mathematical calculations when they are first converted to an equivalent decimal number. Because a percentage is "X out of 100" (e.g. 25% = 25 out of 100), a percentage value is equivalent to "X hundredths" (e.g. 25% = 25 hundredths or 0.25). Therefore, to convert a percentage to its equivalent decimal number value, simply *divide* the number by 100 or "move" the decimal point two places to the *left*. As described in Chapter 2, any trailing zeroes in the most right-hand positions of a decimal number are usually dropped. In addition to the examples shown in Table 4.1, the following percentage conversions also illustrate the concept.

$$1\% = 0.01$$

$$20\% = 0.20 = 0.2$$

$$300\% = 3.00 = 3$$

$$0.5\% = 0.005$$

$$0.037\% = 0.000\,37$$

Table 4.1 Table of conversions between common fractions and the equivalent percentages and decimal numbers

Common fraction	Percentage equivalent	Decimal number equivalent
$\frac{1}{2}$	50%	0.5
$\frac{1}{4}$	25%	0.25
$\frac{3}{4}$	75%	0.75
$\frac{1}{3}$	33.3%	0.333
$\frac{2}{3}$	66% (rounded)	0.667 (rounded)
$\frac{1}{5}$	20%	0.2
$\frac{1}{8}$	12.5%	0.125
$\frac{1}{10}$	10%	0.1

Because percentages were converted to decimal numbers by dividing the number by 100, it is logical to assume that to convert a decimal number back into an equivalent percentage only requires *multiplying* the decimal number by 100 or moving the decimal point two places to the *right* and adding a percent sign.

$$0.15 = 15\%$$

$$0.02 = 2\%$$

$$1.00 = 100\%$$

$$0.0045 = 0.45\%$$

4.3 Conversion of Fractions to Percentages

Common fractions, such as those shown in Table 4.1, should be memorized to facilitate fraction-to-percentage conversions in simple calculations. Otherwise, fractions are converted to percentages by first dividing the fraction as described in Chapter 3 to produce a decimal number, then converting decimal number to the percentage equivalent by moving the decimal point two places to the right. Some examples are shown below:

$$\frac{5}{8} = 5 \div 8 = 0.625, \text{ which is converted to } 62.5\%$$

$$\frac{8}{32} = 8 \div 32 = 0.25, \text{ which is converted to } 25\%$$

4.4 Finding Percentages of a Whole

It is important that the veterinary professional be able to convert written or verbal orders with percentages into the correct mathematical equations to ensure proper calculations or dosage adjustments. Here are several different ways the word "percentage" might be phrased in adjusting a dose:

1) Twenty percent of a 100 mg dose is how many milligrams?
2) How much drug will be given if 75% of the original 100 mg dose is given?
3) How many milligrams are being given when using 120% of the 100 mg dose?
4) What amount of drug is used to increase or decrease a 100 mg dose by 20%?
5) How much of the 200 mg dose is left after 20% is removed?
6) What percentage of 100 mg is 20 mg?
7) Twenty milligrams is what percentage of 100 mg?

Each of these sentences asks something slightly different and requires a different mathematical manipulation of the dose to make the appropriate adjustment.

In the first sentence, "Twenty percent of a 100 mg dose is how many milligrams?" is asking to determine the number of milligrams found in the 20% piece of the whole 100 mg. To identify the quantity of the whole represented by 20%, the whole (100 mg) is multiplied by the "fraction" (20%). The 20% percentage value is converted into its decimal number equivalent which is then multiplied by the whole (100 mg).

$$20\% = 0.20 = 0.2$$

$$0.2 \times 100 \text{ mg} = 20 \text{ mg}$$

At the beginning of this chapter the definition of percentage was given as "the number of items out of 100 items". In the problem above, 20% indeed equals 20 mg (20 items) out of 100 mg (100 items). Therefore, the following general equation can be used to determine the amount of the whole represented by the percentage value (the fractional part of the whole):

whole amount × the percentage = fractional amount in the percentage

For the example just shown, this formula would translate into:

$$100 \, mg \times 0.2 = 20 \, mg$$

In the second sentence of the examples, "How much drug will be given if 75% of the original 100 mg dose is given?", the quantity of the fractional amount (75%) is again identified. Therefore, the same general equation above can be used:

whole amount × the percentage = fractional amount in the percentage

convert percentage to decimal form : 75% = 0.75

$$100 \, mg \times 0.75 = 75 \, mg$$

The third example statement, "How many milligrams are being given when using 120% of the 100 mg dose?" seems to be confusing because the fractional 120% seems to say that it represents "120 items out of 100 items." meaning that the "fractional" part is bigger than the whole (100 mg)! While theoretically one cannot have greater or more than 100% of anything (100% = all = everything = the entire amount, etc.), expressions such as this are commonly used in practice. In this situation the percentage number greater than 100% indicates the resulting fractional amount is going to be greater than 100% or greater than the original whole. In the case of 120%, the amount represented by 120% will be the entire whole amount (100%) plus an additional 20% of the whole.

$$120\% = 100\% + 20\%$$

The answer could be found by adding the whole (100 mg) to the amount found by calculating 20% of the whole (20% of 100 mg). However, instead of doing a multistep calculation, it is easier to convert the 120% into a decimal and multiplying as would be done for a proper percentage number.

$$120\% = 1.20 = 1.2$$

whole amount × the percentage = fractional amount in the percentage

$$100 \, mg \times 1.2 = 120 \, mg$$

Thus, 120% of a 100 mg dose represents a dose that is *increased* from 100 mg to 120 mg.

4.5 Subtracting or Adding the Percentage Fraction of the Whole

The fourth statement in the examples asks a different question than the previous three examples: "What amount of drug is used to increase or decrease a 100 mg dose by 20%?" Unlike the previous examples where the amount or value of the percentage fraction itself was being determined, this question is asking how much of the original whole amount is going to be left after subtraction or addition of the percentage amount. For this problem, the value of the fractional amount must first be determined (as done previously), and then that amount is added or subtracted from the original whole.

To determine "What amount of drug is used to *increase* a 100 mg dose by 20%?" the 20% of 100 mg is first determined as described previously.

$$20\% = 0.20 = 0.2$$

whole amount × the percentage = fractional amount in the percentage

$$100\,mg \times 0.2 = 20\,mg$$

This 20 mg is the amount by which the dose is being increased. So the final dose to be administered would be the original amount plus the 20 mg:

$$100\,mg + 20\,mg = 120\,mg$$

Note that if an amount is being increased by 20%, the same answer would be derived if the 20% were added to the 100% and the resulting 120% (equal to 1.20 or 1.2) be used as the percentage in the formula.

whole amount × the percentage = fractional amount in the percentage

$$100\,mg \times 1.2 = 120\,mg$$

To answer the question of "What amount of drug is used to *decrease* a 100 mg dose by 20%?" the fractional amount of the whole amount would again be determined (100 mg × 20% = 20 mg) and that amount subtracted from the whole amount:

$$100\,mg - 20\,mg = 80\,mg$$

The new dose would be 80 mg after the 100 mg had been decreased by 20%. Note also that if the 20% reduction percentage was mathematically subtracted from 100%, this would give the percentage of 80%, which provides a decimal number (0.80 or 0.8) by which the whole could be multiplied to produce the same answer.

whole amount × the percentage = fractional amount in the percentage

$$100\,mg \times 0.8 = 80\,mg$$

For the fifth statement in the examples, "How much of the 200 mg dose is left after 20% is removed?" the two-step process just described would solve this problem. In this case the whole amount is 200 mg and the amount of drug represented by 20% must first be identified and then that amount removed from 200 mg whole.

whole amount × the percentage = fractional amount in the percentage

$$200\,mg \times 0.2 = 40\,mg$$

$$200\,mg - 40\,mg = 160\,mg \text{ for the new reduced dose}$$

Again, note that this question is asking how much drug would be left over after 20% is removed. Thus, 100% minus 20% equals 80%. 80% of the drug would remain after 20% is removed. Using 0.8 for the percentage in the formula produces the same answer.

whole amount × the percentage = fractional amount in the percentage

$$200\,mg \times 0.8 = 160\,mg$$

4.6 Determining Percentages Represented by the Fractional Component

In statements number 6 and 7 in the examples, the veterinary technician is asked to determine what percentage of the whole is represented by the fractional amount:

6) What percentage of 100 mg is 20 mg?
7) Twenty milligrams is what percentage of 100 mg?

The same general formula can be used to identify the percentage represented by the smaller fractional amount, except instead of knowing the percentage and the amount of the whole, the amount of the whole and the amount of the fractional component are known and the percentage represents the unknown needing to be solved.

whole amount × the percentage = fractional amount in the percentage

$$100\,mg \times \text{the percentage} = 20\,mg$$

Algebraically, the equation is rearranged so that the two known values are on one side of the equal sign and the unknown (the percentage) is on the other. Algebraic rearranging of equations will be discussed in greater detail in Chapter 5. For now, please accept that the rearranged equation becomes this:

$$\text{the percentage} = \frac{\text{fractional amount in the percentage}}{\text{whole amount}}$$

$$\text{the percentage} = \frac{20\,mg}{100\,mg}$$

Because fractions also function as a division problem, the numerator (top number) is divided by the denominator (bottom number) to give the answer as a decimal number. The decimal number is then converted into the equivalent percentage.

$$\text{the percentage} = \frac{20\,mg}{100\,mg} = 0.2 = 0.20 = 20\%$$

Therefore, 20 mg is 20% of 100 mg.

Other examples are shown in Table 4.2 below.

Table 4.2 Calculations needed to determine percentage of fractional component of a whole.

Original statement	Calculation to determine the answer
What percentage of 400 mg is 50 mg?	$\text{percentage} = \dfrac{50\,\text{mg}}{400\,\text{mg}} = 0.125 = 12.5\%$
Twenty-five milligrams is what percentage of 200 mg?	$\text{percentage} = \dfrac{25\,\text{mg}}{200\,\text{mg}} = 0.125 = 12.5\%$
What percentage is 150 mL of 250 mL?	$\text{percentage} = \dfrac{150\,\text{mL}}{250\,\text{mL}} = 0.6 = 60\%$
1.5 mg is what percentage of 10 mg?	$\text{percentage} = \dfrac{1.5\,\text{mg}}{10\,\text{mg}} = 0.15 = 15\%$

By practicing working with percentages on a regular basis, veterinary technicians should be able to convert verbal or written directions to these equations to accurately and efficiently solve dosing problems.

4.7 Chapter 4 Practice Problems

1 Convert the following percentages to decimals:

   A) 50%
   B) 25%
   C) 1.5%
   D) 0.7%
   E) 10.23%
   F) 0.085%
   G) 125%
   H) 203.55%

2 Convert the following decimals to percentages:

   A) 0.75
   B) 0.125
   C) 0.015
   D) 0.0035
   E) 0.10
   F) 0.081 25
   G) 1.25
   H) 3.001

3 Convert the following percentages to fractions, without a calculator:

   A) 50%
   B) 25%
   C) 12.5%
   D) 1.0%
   E) 0.1%
   F) 0.025%

    G) 125.00%

    H) 512.50%

4   Convert the following fractions to percentages:

    A) $\dfrac{1}{2} =$

    B) $\dfrac{3}{4} =$

    C) $\dfrac{1}{8} =$

    D) $\dfrac{1}{32} =$

    E) $\dfrac{1}{10} =$

    F) $\dfrac{2}{5} =$

    G) $\dfrac{9}{32} =$

    H) $\dfrac{24}{56} =$

5   If the veterinary technician is going to increase a dose by 25%, she needs to multiply the dose by what decimal number?

6   The number of tablets to be dispensed to Mr. Jones was decreased by the following equation: "45 tablets × 0.33 = 15 tablets." What percentage is 15 of 45?

7   If you have to "decrease the amount of intravenous fluid by one fourth," by what percentage is the volume of administered fluid decreased?

8   If the veterinary technician is told to "decrease an intravenous dose of drug to 1/10 of the original 250 mg dose," how much drug will be administered?

9   "Fifteen percent of a 200 mg dose of amoxicillin" is how many milligrams? If, instead, the dose was to be decreased by 15%, what would the new dose of amoxicillin be?

10   The dose of some drugs normally metabolized by the liver needs to be reduced by 25% in patients with significant liver disease. If one of these drugs is normally dosed at 120 mg, what would be the new adjusted dose for an animal with liver disease?

11   The veterinarian changed the drug dose from 250 mg to 125 mg. By what percentage was the dose decreased?

12 An animal was on a 25 mg daily dose of prednisone and then the dose was increased to 75 mg a day. What percentage increase in dose is this?

13 An animals was started on an IV treatment with 2000 mL of medication. Four hours later, only 250 mL is left. By what percentage has the original amount been reduced? What percentage of the medication is left to be administered?

14 There is only 10% of the original 30 mL of medication left in a vial. What volume (in mL) is left in the vial? How many milliliters have been removed?

15 The dose of the beta-blocker drug (antiarrhythmia heart drug) being used for a patient in the ICU is currently 200% of what it was 3 days ago. If the original dose was X mg, how would you calculate the current dose based upon the old dose of X mg?

16 Because of a patient's decreased renal function, the calculated 600 mg dose of gentamicin (an antibiotic) needs to be decreased by 12.5%. How much gentamicin (in milligrams) will this animal now be receiving?

17 A dog with epilepsy (seizures) is not well controlled at a dose of 60 mg every 12 hours. The veterinarian decides that the dose should be given at 175% of the current dose. How much drug will this dog receive every 12 hours?

18 Convert each of the following statements into a mathematical equation and solve. For example, "50% of a 200 mg dose is how many milligrams" would translate to "0.5×200 mg" and the answer would be "100 mg."

A) If we use 25% of the original 600 mg dose, how much will be used?
B) How much drug will I give if I want to use 45% of the original 300 mg dose?
C) If I have 200 mg and want to give 75% of the dose, what dose am I giving?
D) How many milligrams are we giving if we use 200% of the 50 mg dose?
E) Twelve and a half milligrams is what percentage of 37.5 mg?
F) We need to increase the amoxicillin dose by 25%. The animal is currently getting 200 mg. How much (in milligrams) is added to the dose? What is the new dose?

5

Review of Key Math Fundamentals

Finding the Unknown *X*

OBJECTIVES

The student will be able to:

1) set up an equation to find the unknown value *X* when given two or three values and their relationship to *X*,
2) perform the mathematical calculations necessary to identify the value of *X*, and
3) apply methods for solving *X* in dose calculations.

In most dose calculations, the veterinary technician is given certain information plus a description of the relationship between the given information and other variables. From this information, a calculation must be created or set up in such a way that a missing value is determined. For example, the given information may be the animal's weight (e.g. 15 kg), the relationship between variables would be a drug *dosage* (e.g. 10 mg/kg of body weight), and the missing value would be the *dose* to be administered to an animal of this weight (e.g. how many milligrams?). It is very important to have a solid grasp of how to accurately set up these equations and to perform the mathematical operations necessary to determine the unknown value *X*.

5.1   Analyzing the Problem and Setting up the Equation

The first step in setting up a calculation to determine the unknown *X* is to identify all of the known values provided by the written or oral instructions, and then determine what constitutes the unknown *X*. For example, the veterinarian orders the compounding (mixing together) of two liquid forms of Drugs A and B into a vial for a specific veterinary patient in the hospital. The veterinarian says to add 12 mL of Drug A to the vial plus 18 mL of Drug B. What will be the volume of the compounded drug?

The known values for this problem are the volume of Drug A (12 mL) and the volume of Drug B (18 mL). The unknown *X* is the final volume, in milliliters. This is a very simple question, but it illustrates the point of properly identifying the known values and the unknown *X* prior to setting up the problem. In more complex problems a greater degree of analysis may be needed to accurately identify the *necessary* known values from the additional unneeded information or values provided.

Once the known values are identified, they are arranged into a mathematical relationship (addition, subtraction, multiplication, division, etc.) on one side of the equal sign in the calculation, placing the unknown *X* by itself on the other side of the equation. The values of the known variables are then plugged into the equation to solve for the unknown *X*.

Medical Mathematics and Dosage Calculations for Veterinary Technicians, Third Edition. Robert Bill.
© 2019 John Wiley & Sons, Inc. Published 2019 by John Wiley & Sons, Inc.
Companion website: www.wiley.com/go/bill/calculations

Drug A + Drug B = total volume in milliliters

12 mL + 18 mL = unknown X in mL

12 mL + 18 mL = 30 mL

The challenge in setting up the problems correctly occurs when the known values and the unknown X do not fall neatly on opposite sides of the equation. For example, the question above might be rephrased as: "Given a total volume of 30 mL from the combined volumes of both Drug A and Drug B, and knowing that Drug A was 12 mL, how much of Drug B must be added to give the correct total volume of 30 mL?" This question would be initially set up as:

Drug A + Drug B = total volume in milliliters

12 mL + unknown X in mL = 30 mL

In this situation the known values and the unknown X are not on opposite sides of the equation. The veterinary technician must then accurately rearrange the equation such that the unknown X is isolated by itself on one side. This rearrangement, which follows basic algebraic principles, is often the source of inaccuracies or miscalculations of doses. Therefore, it is important to review how these mathematical rearrangements are performed to better ensure dose calculations and medical math are accurately performed.

5.2 Addition: Moving Numbers to the Other Side of the Equation

The equal sign acts like the fulcrum or balance point on a scale. Therefore, anything that is done to one side of the equation must be done to the other to maintain the equality (the "balance") between the two sides. If a value of 15 is taken away from one side of an equation, a value of 15 must be removed from the other to maintain the mathematical "balance" of the equation. This concept is used to "move" any known value from one side of the equation to the other side of the equal sign leaving the unknown by itself. In the example used above, the 12 mL volume of Drug A is on the same side as the unknown X, which is the volume of Drug B.

Drug A + Drug B = total volume in milliliters

12 mL + unknown X in mL = 30 mL

To "move" the 12 mL to the same side as the 30 mL and thus isolate the unknown X by itself on one side of the equation, we can add –12 mL to the 12 mL to make it zero.

12 mL – 12 mL + unknown X in mL = 30 mL

0 mL + unknown X in mL = 30 mL

unknown X in mL = 30 mL

But this is an inaccurate representation because whatever is done to one side of the equation, must be done to the other. Therefore, if 12 mL was subtracted from one side, then 12 mL must be subtracted from the other side of the equation.

12 mL – 12 mL + unknown X in mL = 30 mL – 12 mL

0 mL + unknown X in mL = 30 mL – 12 mL

unknown X in mL $= 30\,\text{mL} - 12\,\text{mL}$

unknown X in mL $= 18\,\text{mL}$

The volume for Drug B (the unknown X) is 18 mL. This answer for the unknown X can be easily checked for accuracy by plugging the calculated answer back into the original equation to see if both sides of the equation are indeed equal.

Drug A + Drug B = total volume in milliliters

$12\,\text{mL} + 18\,\text{mL} = 30\,\text{mL}$

$30\,\text{mL} = 30\,\text{mL}$

Note that when moving fractions to properly set up an addition problem with the unknown X isolated on one side, the negative fraction of itself can be added to both sides to "move" the known fraction from one side of the equation to the other side, or the known fraction can be first converted into a decimal number (see Chapter 3) and then the equivalent negative decimal number added to both sides. An example illustrating both methods is shown below.

$$3 + 23 = X + \frac{3}{4}$$

$$3 + 23 = X + 0.75$$

$$3 + 23 - 0.75 = X + 0.75 - 0.75$$

$$3 + 23 - 0.75 = X$$

or

$$3 + 23 = X + \frac{3}{4}$$

$$3 + 23 - \frac{3}{4} = X + \frac{3}{4} - \frac{3}{4}$$

$$3 + 23 - \frac{3}{4} = X$$

5.3 Subtraction: Moving Negative Numbers or a Negative Unknown X

In the example subtraction problem shown below, there is a negative 30 kg ("–30 kg") on the left side of the equation and a negative unknown X ("–X") on the right side of the equation.

$40\,\text{kg} - 30\,\text{kg} = 60\,\text{kg} - X\,\text{kg}$

To solve this problem the unknown X needs to be isolated by itself on one side of the equation by moving all of the known values to the other side of the equation. This can be done by subtracting 60 kg from both sides of the equation, in a similar way to how this was done in the addition problems.

$$40\,kg - 30\,kg = 60\,kg - X\,kg$$

$$40\,kg - 30\,kg - 60\,kg = 60\,kg - 60\,kg - X\,kg$$

$$-50\,kg = -X\,kg$$

The calculation results in a *negative* 50 being equal to a *negative X*. The value for the correct answer is actually *positive* 50. If both sides of the equation are multiplied by –1 the resulting answer would be "50 kg = X kg". To avoid confusion over the positive or negative value of the answer, the equation should be initially set up so that the unknown X is a positive X, not a negative X.

If the original equation has the unknown X being negative, then the unknown negative X needs to be mathematically moved to the other side of the equation by adding a positive X to both sides of the equation. A negative X plus a positive X equals zero, so the negative unknown X "drops out" of that side of the equation and a positive unknown X appears on the other side of the equation. This satisfies the need to set up the equation with a positive unknown X.

$$40\,kg - 30\,kg = 60\,kg - X\,kg$$

$$40\,kg - 30\,kg + X\,kg = 60\,kg - X\,kg + X\,kg$$

$$40\,kg - 30\,kg + X\,kg = 60\,kg$$

To complete the set up for calculating the answer, the rest of the known values (40 kg and –30 kg) can be moved to the right side of the equation by adding a negative 40 ("–40") and a positive 30 to both sides of the equation to "neutralize" to zero the known values on the left side of the equation, leaving just the positive unknown X isolated by itself on the left side. All of the known values are now separated from the positive unknown X.

$$40\,kg - 40\,kg - 30\,kg + 30\,kg + X\,kg = 60\,kg - 40\,kg + 30\,kg$$

$$0\,kg - 0\,kg + X\,kg = 60\,kg - 40\,kg + 30\,kg$$

$$X\,kg = 60\,kg - 40\,kg + 30\,kg$$

The calculation can now be performed.

$$X\,kg = 60\,kg - 40\,kg + 30\,kg$$

$$X\,kg = 20\,kg + 30\,kg$$

$$X\,kg = 50\,kg$$

Note that the actual value of X after a different calculation might be a negative number (e.g. $X = -20$), but during the equation set up, the unknown X needs to be arranged so it is represented as a positive X.

The answer is checked by plugging it into the original equation to see if both sides of the equation are the same.

$$40\,\text{kg} - 30\,\text{kg} = 60\,\text{kg} - X\,\text{kg}$$

$$40\,\text{kg} - 30\,\text{kg} = 60\,\text{kg} - 50\,\text{kg}$$

$$10\,\text{kg} = 10\,\text{kg}$$

Both sides of the equation are balanced and equal each other so the answer must have been correct.

Thus, the three essential steps to set up and solve for unknown X in addition and subtraction problems are:

1) rearrange the equation, if necessary, to make the unknown X *positive,*
2) isolate the positive unknown X on one side of the equation, and
3) perform the mathematical operation on the rearranged equation.

Using these same three steps, problems containing a mixture of positive and negative values can be consistently and accurately solved. For example, a veterinary technician was creating a mixture of Drug A and Drug B to be mixed in water for oral administration. The drug dose called for 250 mg of a powdered Drug A to be added to 40 mg of a second powdered Drug B. However, the veterinarian wanted to reduce the amount of Drug A by 15 mg and reduce the amount of Drug B by some unknown X amount so that the total combined amount of Drug A and Drug B was exactly 265 mg. Although this sounds complicated, by breaking the information down into parts, the veterinary technician was able to construct the following calculation:

$$\text{Original amount of Drug A} = 250\,\text{mg}$$

Need to decrease Drug A by 15 mg

$$\text{New amount of Drug A} = 250\,\text{mg} - 15\,\text{mg}$$

$$\text{Original amount of Drug B} = 40\,\text{mg}$$

Need to decrease Drug B by unknown X mg

$$\text{New amount of Drug B} = 40\,\text{mg} - X\,\text{mg}$$

This total of the two compounds had to total 265 mg.

$$\text{Drug A (new)} + \text{Drug B (new)} = 265\,\text{mg}$$

$$(250\,\text{mg} - 15\,\text{mg}) + (40\,\text{mg} - X\,\text{mg}) = 265\,\text{mg}$$

$$250\,\text{mg} - 15\,\text{mg} + 40\,\text{mg} - X\,\text{mg} = 265\,\text{mg}$$

The unknown X value in the equation is a negative unknown X, so it needs to be moved to the other side of the equation to make it a positive unknown X.

$$250\,\text{mg} - 15\,\text{mg} + 40\,\text{mg} - X\,\text{mg} = 265\,\text{mg}$$

$$250\,\text{mg} - 15\,\text{mg} + 40\,\text{mg} - X\,\text{mg} + X\,\text{mg} = 265\,\text{mg} + X\,\text{mg}$$

$$250\,\text{mg} - 15\,\text{mg} + 40\,\text{mg} = 265\,\text{mg} + X\,\text{mg}$$

Now the positive unknown value X must be isolated to one side of the equation by itself by moving the 265 mg to the other side of the equation.

$$250\,\text{mg} - 15\,\text{mg} + 40\,\text{mg} = 265\,\text{mg} + X\,\text{mg}$$

$$250\,\text{mg} - 15\,\text{mg} + 40\,\text{mg} - 265\,\text{mg} = 265\,\text{mg} - 265\,\text{mg} + X\,\text{mg}$$

$$250\,\text{mg} - 15\,\text{mg} + 40\,\text{mg} - 265\,\text{mg} = X\,\text{mg}$$

$$235\,\text{mg} + 40\,\text{mg} - 265\,\text{mg} = X\,\text{mg}$$

$$275\,\text{mg} - 265\,\text{mg} = 10\,\text{mg} = X\,\text{mg}$$

Remember that X mg is the amount to be removed from Drug B.

Check your answer by plugging the solution into the original equation:

$$250\,\text{mg} - 15\,\text{mg} + 40\,\text{mg} - X\,\text{mg} = 265\,\text{mg}$$

$$250\,\text{mg} - 15\,\text{mg} + 40\,\text{mg} - 10\,\text{mg} = 265\,\text{mg}$$

$$235\,\text{mg} + 30\,\text{mg} = 265\,\text{mg}$$

$$265\,\text{mg} = 265\,\text{mg}$$

The values are the same on both sides of the equation; therefore, the answer must be correct. By remembering and applying the three essential steps in solving for the unknown X, even relatively complex equations can be solved.

Note that fractions in unknown X subtraction problems are handled using the same techniques used for fractions in the addition problems (Section 5.2).

5.4 Finding the Unknown X in Multiplication Problems

The vast majority of dosage calculations require the veterinary professional to solve for the unknown X in a multiplication or division type of problem. Therefore, the unknown X must still be isolated to one side of the equation by applying basic algebraic rules.

If you are given three known values in a multiplication problem and then asked to find a fourth unknown X value, two of the previously listed three steps for addition and subtraction problems are used:

1) Isolate the positive unknown X on one side of the equation.
2) Perform the mathematical operation on the rearranged equation.

Unlike in addition and subtraction problems where it was very important to set up the problem with the unknown X being a positive unknown X before the problem was calculated, this is not as much of a concern with multiplication or division problems. Often in multiplication or division problems the resulting answer value can still result in the answer being equal to a negative unknown X. The negative unknown X in the answer still needs to be converted to a positive unknown X to reflect the accurate value in the answer, but this conversion of a negative unknown X to a positive unknown X is simple and can occur after the calculation is completed. For example, if a multiplication problem was solved to give the value of the answer (positive 35) equal to a negative unknown X.

$$35 = -X$$

To identify the correct value for the answer, the negative unknown X must be converted to a positive unknown X. In this case, the negative unknown X was converted to a positive unknown X by multiplying both sides of the equation by -1. This is based on the mathematical rule that any negative number multiplied by another negative number results a positive number:

$$35 = -X$$

$$35 \times -1 = -X \times -1$$

$$-35 = X$$

Once the negative unknown X has been converted to a positive unknown X, the true value of the answer (-35) is revealed.

Let's illustrate the application of multiplication to solve for the unknown X by using a clinical example. Mrs. Smith's dog was dispensed thirty-five 100 mg tablets and she was instructed to give one tablet daily. However, because it is so difficult to administer a pill to her dog, Mrs. Smith prefers giving her dog smaller-sized tablets. To improve the likelihood of Mrs. Smith complying with the need to give the medication daily, the veterinarian gave new drug orders to dispense a bottle of 50 mg tablets at the dose of two 50 mg tablets once daily. If Mrs. Smith had originally been dispensed 35 of the 100 mg tablets (35 days' worth of medication), how many 50 mg tablets would need to be dispensed to give Mrs. Smith 35 days' worth of medication?

Although this problem can be readily solved in your head without a calculator, setting up the problem illustrates how to organize the equation to arrive at the correct answer. In this problem the old dose using 100 mg tablets has to equal the new dose using 50 mg tablets. Thus, the old dose should be on one side of the equation and the new dose on the other side of the equation, since they must equal each other.

$$\text{old dose} = \text{new dose}$$

$$100\,\text{mg} \times 35\,\text{tablets} = 50\,\text{mg} \times X\,\text{tablets}$$

Just as was done in addition or subtraction problems, any number on the same side as the unknown X has to be moved to the other side of the equation to isolate the unknown X on one side of the equation by itself. In addition or subtraction problems this was done by "neutralizing" the value of numbers to zero by adding the negative of the number to both sides of the equation. However, in multiplication or division problems, a number is "neutralized" and moved to the other side of the equation by making it have the value of 1 using the mathematical rule than any number multiplied or divided by 1 equals that same number.

As stated in Chapter 3, the way any number is made into the value of 1 is by multiplying it by its reciprocal. In this problem, the 50 mg is converted to 1 by multiplying by its reciprocal (1/50). Of course the other side of the equation must also be multiplied by 1/50. This results in the unknown X on the right side being multiplied by 1 and the values on other side of the equation being multiplied by the same 1/50 number. Since 1 multiplied by the unknown X equals the unknown X, the unknown X in this example problem is now isolated on one side of the equation.

$$100\,mg \times 35\,tablets = 50\,mg \times X\,tablets$$

$$100\,mg \times \frac{1}{50\,mg} \times 35\,tablets = 50\,mg \times \frac{1}{50\,mg} \times X\,tablets$$

$$100\,mg \times \frac{1}{50\,mg} \times 35\,tablets = 1 \times X\,tablets$$

$$100\,mg \times \frac{1}{50\,mg} \times 35\,tablets = X\,tablets$$

The problem is now set up so that it meets the first criteria of having the unknown X isolated on one side of the equation and the problem can now be calculated.

$$100\,mg \times \frac{1}{50\,mg} \times 35\,tablets = X\,tablets$$

$$\frac{100\,mg}{50\,mg} \times 35\,tablets = X\,tablets$$

$$2 \times 35\,tablets = X\,tablets$$

$$70\,tablets = X\,tablets$$

The answer indicates that 70 of the 50 mg tablets should be dispensed to be equivalent to the 35 of the 100 mg tablets. Check the validity of the answer by plugging the answer into the original equation:

$$100\,mg \times 35\,tablets = 50\,mg \times X\,tablets$$

$$100\,mg \times 35\,tablets = 50\,mg \times 70\,tablets$$

$$350 = 350$$

When there are fractions in a multiplication problem, the same basic techniques used previously are employed to isolate the unknown X on one side of the equation. Here is an example problem:

$$2 \times 3 = \frac{3}{4} \times X$$

To isolate the unknown X on the right side of the equation, the 3/4 is changed into a value of 1 by multiplying it and the other side of the equation by its reciprocal, 4/3.

$$2 \times 3 = \frac{3}{4} \times X$$

$$2 \times 3 \times \frac{4}{3} = \frac{3}{4} \times \frac{4}{3} \times X$$

$$2 \times 3 \times \frac{4}{3} = 1 \times X$$

$$2 \times 3 \times \frac{4}{3} = X$$

Once set up correctly with the unknown X isolated to one side, the equation is solved by multiplication of fractions and whole numbers as discussed in Chapter 3. In this case, the 3 in the denominator of the 4/3 improper fraction can be reduced with the whole number 3 to produce a simpler equation to calculate:

$$2 \times \cancel{3} \times \frac{4}{\cancel{3}} = X$$

$$2 \times 1 \times \frac{4}{1} = X$$

$$2 \times 1 \times 4 = X$$

$$8 = X$$

Plugging the answer back into the original equation verifies that this is the correct answer:

$$2 \times 3 = \frac{3}{4} \times X$$

$$2 \times 3 = \frac{3}{4} \times 8$$

$$2 \times 3 = \frac{3}{1} \times 2$$

$$2 \times 3 = 3 \times 2$$

$$6 = 6$$

For mixed numbers (whole numbers and fractions together), the mixed numbers can be converted into improper fractions, then converted to 1 using the reciprocal to "move" the mixed number to the other side of the equation, isolating the unknown X as described for the previous problem.

$$3 \times 4 = 1\frac{1}{2} \times X$$

$$3 \times 4 = \frac{3}{2} \times X$$

$$3 \times 4 \times \frac{2}{3} = \frac{3}{2} \times \frac{2}{3} \times X$$

$$3 \times 4 \times \frac{2}{3} = 1 \times X$$

$$3 \times 4 \times \frac{2}{3} = X$$

simplified: $3 \times 4 \times \dfrac{2}{3} = X$

$$1 \times 4 \times \dfrac{2}{1} = X$$

$$4 \times 2 = X$$

$$8 = X$$

Check the answer for accuracy by plugging the answer into the original equation:

$$3 \times 4 = 1\dfrac{1}{2} \times X$$

$$3 \times 4 = 1\dfrac{1}{2} \times 8$$

$$3 \times 4 = \dfrac{3}{2} \times 8$$

$$3 \times 4 = \dfrac{3}{1} \times 4$$

$$3 \times 4 = 3 \times 4$$

$$12 = 12$$

Another example illustrates these concepts and incorporates the principles from Chapter 3 for working with a mixture of multiplication of fractions and decimal to fraction conversions.

Solve the following: $0.25 \times 5 \times 8 = 2 \times \dfrac{1}{10} \times X$

Isolate the unknown X to one side by using the reciprocals of 2 and 1/10.

$$0.25 \times 5 \times 8 \times \dfrac{1}{2} \times 10 = 2 \times \dfrac{1}{2} \times \dfrac{1}{10} \times 10 \times X$$

$$0.25 \times 5 \times 8 \times \dfrac{1}{2} \times 10 = 1 \times 1 \times X$$

$$0.25 \times 5 \times 8 \times \dfrac{1}{2} \times 10 = X$$

The equation is now set up to perform the calculation. Based upon the principles in Chapter 3, the fraction 1/2 can be changed to the decimal 0.5, or "8 × 1/2" can be reduced to "4 × 1," or the product of all the numerators (the non-fractioned numbers and the top part of any fraction) multiplied can be divided by 2. Each of these techniques would give the same answer. The three possible methods to find the solution are shown below:

- converting the fraction to a decimal

$$0.25 \times 5 \times 8 \times \frac{1}{2} \times 10 = X$$

  which converts to $0.25 \times 5 \times 8 \times 0.5 \times 10 = X$

- using a simplified fraction

$$0.25 \times 5 \times 4 \times \frac{1}{1} \times 10 = X$$

  which converts to $0.25 \times 5 \times 4 \times 10 = X$

- or with all numerators over all denominators

$$\frac{0.25 \times 5 \times 8 \times 1 \times 10}{2} = X$$

  which coverts to $\frac{100}{2} = X$

All these then give $50 = X$.

Check this by plugging the answer into the original equation to see if the equation balances.

$$0.25 \times 5 \times 8 = 2 \times \frac{1}{10} \times X$$

$$0.25 \times 5 \times 8 = 2 \times \frac{1}{10} \times 50$$

$$0.25 \times 40 = \frac{2}{10} \times 50$$

$$10 = \frac{100}{10}$$

$$10 = 10$$

5.5   When the Unknown *X* is in the Denominator

Although in multiplication and division problems you do not have to adjust the equation setup to insure the unknown X is positive, you do have to make sure the initial equation is set up so that the unknown X is always in the numerator (the top part of the fraction). On occasions, especially with division problems discussed in

Section 5.6, the unknown X can end up as a denominator (on the bottom of the fraction), such as when the problem is set up as shown below.

$$\frac{20}{5} = 2 \times \frac{36}{X}$$

If this equation was not rearranged to get the X into the numerator position before calculating, the answer would be expressed as $1/X$ instead of X. The actual correct value of the answer would then have to be calculated by dividing 1 by the value of X.

Fortunately, the same principle of reciprocal multiplication can be employed to rearrange the location of the unknown X from denominator into the numerator and insure that the equation is set up with the unknown X in the numerator before performing the calculation. In the problem above, both sides of the equation are multiplied by the reciprocal of $1/X$, which would be $X/1$ (or just X), resulting in the X becoming a numerator ($X/1$ or X) on the other side of the equation.

$$\frac{20}{5} = 2 \times \frac{36}{X}$$

$$\frac{20}{5} \times \frac{X}{1} = 2 \times \frac{36}{X} \times \frac{X}{1}$$

$$\frac{20}{5} \times X = 2 \times \frac{36}{1}$$

$$\frac{20}{5} \times X = 2 \times 36$$

Now that the unknown X is properly located in the numerator position, the unknown X can be isolated to one side of the equation by multiplying the reciprocal of the number needing to be moved.

$$\frac{20}{5} \times X = 2 \times 36$$

$$\frac{20}{5} \times \frac{5}{20} \times X = 2 \times 36 \times \frac{5}{20}$$

$$1 \times X = 2 \times 36 \times \frac{5}{20}$$

$$X = 2 \times 36 \times \frac{5}{20}$$

The problem is now in the proper form (unknown X is isolated and unknown X is in the numerator) and ready to be solved. As with any fraction multiplication problem, the problem should be simplified before calculating, to make it easier to solve. One possible simplification is shown below.

$$X = 2 \times 36 \times \frac{5}{20}$$

$$X = 1 \times 36 \times \frac{5}{10}$$

$$X = 1 \times 18 \times \frac{5}{5}$$

$$X = 1 \times 18 \times 1$$

$$X = 18$$

Check the answer by plugging it into the original problem to see if both sides of the equation have equal values:

$$\frac{20}{5} = 2 \times \frac{36}{X}$$

$$\frac{20}{5} = 2 \times \frac{36}{18}$$

$$\frac{20}{5} = 2 \times 2$$

$$\frac{4}{1} = 2 \times 2$$

$$4 = 4$$

To summarize, the steps for multiplication are:

1) Make sure the unknown X is in the numerator (top part of a fraction).
2) Isolate the positive unknown X on one side of the equation.
3) Perform the mathematical operation on the rearranged equation.

Now that the principles of how to accurately perform multiplication problems to solve for the unknown X have been discussed, the general methods by which these problems are solved when using a calculator are shown in Table 5.1.

Table 5.1 Steps for solving multiplication equations for unknown X

Form of the original problem	Steps to solve for X using a calculator
$A \times B = X \times C$	1) multiply A by B 2) divide answer from step 1 by C
$A \times B = C \times X$	1) multiply A by B 2) divide answer from step 1 by C
$A \times X = B \times C$	1) multiply B by C 2) divide answer from step 1 by A
$X \times A = B \times C$	1) multiply B by C 2) divide answer from step 1 by A

5.6   Finding the Unknown *X* in Division Problems

Setting up a division problem involves the same three steps described above to solve multiplication problems. However, there are three additional basic mathematical rules from Chapter 3 that are more frequently utilized in division problems:

1) Fractions can be converted to a decimal number by dividing the numerator (top number of fraction) by the denominator (bottom number of fraction). Therefore, any number that needs to be divided by another number can be expressed in an equation as a fraction where the numerator is the number that must be divided and the denominator is the number of parts into which the numerator value must be split. (e.g. 1/2 is the value of one that is to be divided into two parts.)
2) Any fraction with a 1 in the denominator has the same value as the numerator (e.g. 20/1 is the same value as 20)

For example, the division problem below can be expressed as two fractions wherein the numerator is the number to be divided and the denominator being the number by which the numerator is being divided.

$$45 \div 15 = X \div 25$$

is equivalent to $\dfrac{45}{15} = \dfrac{X}{25}$

To solve this problem for the unknown X, the rules employed in the multiplication problems can be used here. First, the unknown X needs to be located in the numerator. In this example, the unknown X is already located in the numerator of the fraction $X/25$. The second step is to isolate the unknown X to one side using the reciprocal method employed with multiplication problems. To "neutralize" the 25 and "move" it to the other side of the equation, both sides of the equation are multiplied by the reciprocal of 1/25 which would be 25/1 or 25.

$$\frac{45}{15} = \frac{X}{25}$$

$$\frac{45}{15} \times \frac{25}{1} = \frac{X}{25} \times \frac{25}{1}$$

$$\frac{45}{15} \times 25 = \frac{X}{25} \times 25$$

$$\frac{45}{15} \times 25 = \frac{X}{1} \times 1$$

$$\frac{45}{15} \times 25 = X$$

Now that the unknown X is isolated and in the numerator position ("X" is the same as "$X/1$"), the problem can be solved. In this case the fraction in the problem can be simplified by dividing 45 and 15 by 15 (done when calculating by hand), or, when performed with a calculator, all the numerators (45 and 25) can be multiplied together then divided by all the denominators (15) multiplied together. Both methods are shown below.

$$\frac{45}{15} \times 25 = X$$

$$\frac{3}{1} \times 25 = X$$

$$3 \times 25 = X$$

$$75 = X$$

or (if done using a calculator)

$$\frac{45}{15} \times 25 = X$$

$$\frac{45 \times 25}{15} = X$$

$$\frac{1125}{15} = X$$

$$75 = X$$

Check it:

$$45 \div 15 = X \div 25$$

$$45 \div 15 = 75 \div 25$$

$$3 = 3$$

Thus, division problems involving an unknown X can be said to have one additional step at the beginning of its process:

1) Convert the whole numbers being divided into fractions (for ease of manipulation).
2) Make sure the unknown X is in the numerator (top part of a fraction).
3) Isolate the positive unknown X on one side of the equation.
4) Perform the mathematical operation on the rearranged equation.

Now that the principles of how to accurately perform division problems to solve for the unknown X have been discussed, the general methods by which these problems are solved when using a calculator are shown in Table 5.2. Notice how the position of unknown X in the problem dictates whether the answer from the first step is multiplied or divided in the second step.

5.7 Unknown *X* Involving Division of Fractions

What about circumstances in which a fraction is involved in the division problem?

$$30 \div 5 = X \div \frac{1}{2}$$

It might seem that one approach would be to isolate the unknown X by multiplying both sides by the reciprocal of 1/2 which would be 2. However, if both sides are multiplied by 2, each individual element of the problem must be multiplied by 2.

Table 5.2 Steps for solving division equations for unknown X

Form of the original problem	Steps to solve for X using a calculator
$A \div B = X \div C$	1) divide A by B 2) multiply C by the answer from step 1
$A \div B = C \div X$	1) divide A by B 2) divide C by the answer from step 1
$A \div X = B \div C$	1) divide B by C 2) divide A by the answer from step 1
$X \div A = B \div C$	1) divide B by C 2) multiply A by the answer from step 1

$$30 \div 5 = X \div \frac{1}{2}$$

$$2 \times (30 \div 5) = 2 \times \left(X \div \frac{1}{2} \right)$$

$$(2 \times 30) \div (2 \times 5) = (2 \times X) \div \left(2 \times \frac{1}{2} \right)$$

$$(60) \div (10) = (2 \times X) \div (1)$$

$$6 = 2 \times X$$

$$6 \times \frac{1}{2} = 2 \times \frac{1}{2} \times X$$

$$3 = X$$

It would be fairly easy to make a mistake when doing this conversion. So an easier approach would be to first convert each fraction to its decimal equivalent and then to proceed as was done in the problems in Section 5.7. As discussed in Chapter 3, the fraction 1/2 is converted to its decimal equivalent of 0.5 by dividing 1 by 2. This fraction is also one of the simple fractions listed in Chapter 3 that all veterinary technicians should know the decimal equivalent without calculating.

$$30 \div 5 = X \div \frac{1}{2}$$

$$30 \div 5 = X \div 0.5$$

Even though the presence of a decimal number in a fraction looks odd, it is perfectly acceptable for helping to perform a calculation properly. First, the division problem is converted into fractions:

$$30 \div 5 = X \div 0.5$$

$$\frac{30}{5} = \frac{X}{0.5}$$

Next, the unknown X value is checked to make sure it is located in the numerator. It is, so the unknown X can be isolated on the right side of the equation. To do so, multiply both sides of the equation by the reciprocal of the number needing to move, just as was done in the previous problems. To remove the 0.5 from the denominator and leave the unknown X by itself, both sides are multiplied by the reciprocal of "1/0.5" which would be 0.5.

$$\frac{30}{5} = \frac{X}{0.5}$$

$$\frac{30}{5} \times 0.5 = \frac{X}{0.5} \times 0.5$$

$$\frac{30}{5} \times 0.5 = \frac{X}{1} \times 1$$

$$\frac{30}{5} \times 0.5 = X$$

Once the unknown X is isolated, the problem is then ready to be solved.

$$\frac{30}{5} \times 0.5 = X$$

$$6 \times 0.5 = X$$

$$3 = X$$

Mathematically this second method of converting fractions into decimal numbers is far more straightforward and less prone to mathematical calculation errors than the method wherein groups of numbers must be multiplied by reciprocals to isolate the unknown X to one side of the equation.

The answer still needs to be checked by plugging it into the original equation to see if both sides of the equation are equal:

$$30 \div 5 = X \div \frac{1}{2}$$

$$30 \div 5 = 3 \div \frac{1}{2}$$

Remember that when a number is divided by a fraction, it is actually multiplied by its reciprocal.

$$30 \div 5 = 6$$

$$6 = 6$$

The steps for solving these types of problems with a calculator are the same as described in Table 5.2 in Section 5.6, except that there is the additional step of converting any fractions into their decimal equivalent before performing the steps described.

Division fractions for solving the unknown X are frequently used in dose calculations but represent some of the trickier mathematical rules. By practicing and mastering the mathematical principles by which the values on either side of the equation can legitimately be moved and by following the essential steps related to isolation of unknown X, the veterinary professional should be able to perform the wide variety of dose calculations that will be presented in the next chapters.

5.8   Chapter 5 Practice Problems

1   Solve for the unknown X in each of the following addition problems:

A) $23 + 5 = X + 13$
B) $X + 56.4 + 261.5 = 62.3 + 573.2$
C) $0.32 + X + 0.021 = 0.5233 + 0.0901$
D) $25 + 6 + 9 = 1/2 + X$
E) $5/6 + X = 63 + 1/6$
F) $100 \text{ mL} + 250 \text{ mL} = X \text{ mL} + 300 \text{ mL}$
G) $34 \text{ mg} + X \text{ mg} = 74 \text{ mg} + 28 \text{ mg}$
H) $X \text{ L} + 2.31 \text{ L} = 7.09 \text{ L} + 1.39 \text{ L}$
I) $0.034 \text{ g} + 0.002 \text{ g} = 0.009 \text{ g} + X \text{ g}$
J) $3/4 \text{ kg} + X \text{ kg} + 2/3 \text{ kg} = 5/12 \text{ kg} + 1/4 \text{ kg}$

2   Solve for the unknown X in each of the following subtraction problems:

A) $12 - 5 = X - 10$
B) $X - 154 = 214 - 23$
C) $5.2 - X = 7.9 - 2.2$
D) $X - 1/6 = 34 - 2/3$
E) $1/3 - 1/12 = 4/6 - X$
F) $45 \text{ gr} - 7.5 \text{ gr} = X \text{ gr} - 37.5 \text{ gr}$
G) $278 \text{ mg} - 32.5 \text{ mg} = 302.5 \text{ mg} - X \text{ mg}$
H) $X \text{ gr} - 15 \text{ gr} = 90 \text{ gr} - 37.5 \text{ gr}$
I) $0.025 \text{ mcg} - X \text{ mcg} = 0.09 \text{ mcg} - 0.0763 \text{ mcg}$
J) $2/3 \text{ kg} - X \text{ kg} = 3/4 \text{ kg} - 7/24 \text{ kg}$

3   Solve for the unknown X in each of the following multiplication problems:

A) $2.5 \times 4.5 = X \times 2.25$
B) $X \times 74.123 = 10.2 \times 12.76$
C) $\dfrac{1}{2} \times \dfrac{3}{4} = X \times \dfrac{7}{8}$
D) $\dfrac{7}{8} \times X = \dfrac{6}{9} \times \dfrac{5}{6}$
E) $X \times \dfrac{5}{12} = \dfrac{13}{24} \times \dfrac{2}{3} \times \dfrac{4}{3}$
F) $\dfrac{16}{12} \times \dfrac{2}{3} = \dfrac{24}{15} \times X$

G) $\dfrac{13}{26} \times \dfrac{5}{3} = X \times \dfrac{4}{3} \times 6$

H) $1\dfrac{2}{3} \times 3\dfrac{1}{6} = X \times 5\dfrac{1}{12}$

I) $X \times 14\dfrac{3}{8} = 0.4 \times 3\dfrac{5}{7}$

J) $-2 \times \dfrac{4}{15} = 4\dfrac{4}{5} \times X \times 0.125$

4   Solve for the unknown X in each of the following division problems:

A) $6.5 \div 4.2 = X \div 3.8$

B) $X \div 7.45 = 1.243 \div 0.25$

C) $8.23 \div X = 7.97 \div 0.01$

D) $13.78 \div 4.223 = 32.31 \div X$

E) $\dfrac{3}{4} \div \dfrac{1}{2} = X \div \dfrac{5}{8}$

F) $X \div \dfrac{2}{3} = \dfrac{3}{12} \div \dfrac{1}{8}$

G) $\dfrac{18}{24} \div X = \dfrac{9}{32} \div \dfrac{1}{16}$

H) $\dfrac{96}{32} \div \dfrac{3}{2} = \dfrac{24}{18} \div X$

I) $2\dfrac{1}{4} \div 1\dfrac{1}{8} = X \div 3\dfrac{1}{16}$

J) $0.02 \div 3\dfrac{3}{8} = X \div 12\dfrac{3}{4}$

5   A pharmacist puts 3 mL of one liquid in a graduated cylinder, to which he adds 12 mL of another liquid. If the pharmacist then puts 5.75 mL in another graduated cylinder, how much of a second liquid would he have to add to the second graduated cylinder to equal the volume of the two liquids in the first graduated cylinder?

6   A veterinarian calculates that a patient needs a total of 240 mg of drug. What fraction of the a vial containing 360 mg of drug would be needed to provide 240 mg dose?

7   An epileptic dog has been receiving phenobarbital to control his seizures as a combination of one 7.5 mg tablet and one 45 mg tablet. The veterinarian wants to switch to a 30 mg tablet, but this won't be enough to be equivalent to the previous dose. How many more milligrams must be added to the 30 mg tablet dose to achieve a dose that is equivalent to the original dose?

Section II

Understanding Units and Labels

6

Measurements Used in Veterinary Medicine

OBJECTIVES

The student will be able to

1) define a given metric unit relative to other metric units of measure (e.g. grams compared to kilograms);
2) accurately communicate numerical values and appropriate abbreviations for metric, apothecary, and household measurements used in veterinary medicine, both orally and in writing;
3) carry out simple key metric conversions to apothecary, household, or avoirdupois measurements used in veterinary medicine;
4) perform basic dosage calculations using the proportion or cancel-out method; and
5) make accurate estimations of dosage calculations without using a calculator.

Different cultures evolved different methods by which to measure length, weight, and volume. Today, some of these measurements are still used in cooking recipes, for distances used in sports, and in medical calculations. Unfortunately, the units of length, volume, and mass (weight) that are used for everyday purposes such as cooking and sports are sometimes cumbersome to use in the medical area. Therefore, units of measurement in the medical field are typically expressed as *metric units* (e.g. kilograms, milliliters, centimeters).

Even though the metric system dominates medical measurements, other unit measurement systems can occasionally be seen in dosage calculations or descriptions of drug amounts. There are apothecary units, such as grains and drams, household units, such as teaspoons, cups, and quarts, and avoirdupois units, which include ounces and pounds. Thus, it is important that the veterinary professional become familiar with the proper use of the measurement systems used in veterinary medicine, and how to convert between units within each system and between different measurement systems.

6.1 Metric Units: The Basics

The metric system is widely used in medical and scientific fields across the world because of its simplicity. While it is not necessary to understand all components of the metric system, it is important to understand how the system is set up and how to convert between different units within the metric system.

The metric system contains three basic units of measurement: *meter* for length, *liter* for volume, and *gram* for mass. Prefixes are added to each of the basic metric units to denote what power of 10 (e.g. 10, 100, 1/10, 1/1000) the unit represents. For example, adding the prefix "kilo" to each of these metric unit bases means to multiply the basic unit by 1000. The commonly used prefixes in the metric system are shown in Table 6.1.

Medical Mathematics and Dosage Calculations for Veterinary Technicians, Third Edition. Robert Bill.
© 2019 John Wiley & Sons, Inc. Published 2019 by John Wiley & Sons, Inc.
Companion website: www.wiley.com/go/bill/calculations

Table 6.1 Commonly used prefixes in the metric system

Prefix	Multiply the base by this	Symbol	English word
tera-	1 000 000 000 or 10^{12}	T	trillion
giga-	1 000 000 000 or 10^9	G	billion
mega-	1 000 000 or 10^6	M	million
kilo-	1000 or 10^3	k	thousand
hector-	100 or 10^2	h	hundred
deka-	10 or 10^1	da	ten
—	1 or 10^0	—	one
deci-	$\frac{1}{10}$ or 0.1 or 10^{-1}	d	tenth
centi-	$\frac{1}{100}$ or 0.01 or 10^{-2}	c	hundredth
milli-	$\frac{1}{1\,000}$ or 0.001 or 10^{-3}	m	thousandth
micro-	$\frac{1}{1\,000\,000}$ or 0.000 001 or 10^{-6}	mc *or* μ	millionth
nano-	$\frac{1}{1\,000\,000\,000}$ or 0.000 000 001 or 10^{-9}	n	billionth
pico-	0.000 000 000 001 or 10^{-12}	p	trillionth
femto-	0.000 000 000 000 001 or 10^{-15}	f	quadrillionth

The larger prefixes, tera-, giga-, and mega-, are commonly used to describe aspects of computers or information transfer rates over the Internet, such as "1 terabyte hard drive," "10 gigabyte flash drive," or "150 megabytes per second." The very small values are often used in veterinary medicine to describe the amount of a drug in the body (e.g. "35 nanograms of digoxin per unit of blood"), a value from a blood test, a microscopic length of a bacterium or parasite egg (e.g. "a 3.1 micrometer egg"), or the concentration of poison in the blood (e.g. "45 picograms of botulism toxin per unit of body weight").

Of this list of prefixes, the ones most commonly used in dosage calculations include kilo-, centi-, milli-, and micro-, of which only kilo- indicates an amount greater than the base unit of 1. All the other prefixes indicate a smaller fractional amount. Therefore, in memorizing these four particular units, remember that a kilo unit is the one that is larger than the base unit, and all the rest are smaller.

As shown in Table 6.1, each metric prefix has a specific abbreviation. Note that when the Greek letter mu, "μ," for "micro-" is handwritten, it can look very similar to a lower case script-written "m" with pointed "peaks." Therefore, the "mc" designation for micro- is being used more commonly in handwritten dosing orders to avoid confusion. However, the "μ" is still often used in printed text.

When referring to more than one metric unit (e.g. 300 kg), an "s" is not added to the abbreviation. So, 300 kilograms would be "300 kg," not "300 kgs." Additional rules for standard writing and pronunciation of metric units are shown in Table 6.2.

6.2 Metric Units of Weight and Mass

Although the terms "mass" and "weight" mean different things in physics, they are often used interchangeably in common clinical language. An animal has a mass of 10 kg, but it weighs 10 kg on the scale, reflecting the

Table 6.2 Rules for writing and speaking in metric units

Rules from the National Institute of Standards and Technology, an agency of the US Department of Commerce. (www.nist.gov)

1) The names of metric units (e.g. "grams," "meters," "milliliter") all start with a lower case letter except at the beginning of a sentence. The exception is "degree Celsius" or "degree Fahrenheit" in which the word "degree" is not capitalized, but the word "Celsius" or "Fahrenheit" is.

2) The abbreviations for metric units (e.g. "g," "m," "kg") are written in lower case *except* for liter (e.g. "mL," "L") and for those units derived from a person's name (e.g. "W" for watt, "Pa" for pascal, "F" for Fahrenheit). Note that the fully written out metric units for liter, watt, and pascal are not capitalized (e.g. in the "mL" abbreviation the "liter" is capitalized but when written out as "milliliter" the "liter" is not capitalized).

3) Metric prefixes that mean a million or more are capitalized (e.g. "M" for mega, "G" for giga) and those less than a million are lower case (e.g. "m" for milli or thousandths, "c" for centi or hundredths).

4) The names of base metric units (e.g. "meter," "gram," "liter") are made plural *only* when the numerical value that precedes them is greater than 1. For example, it is "0.5 meter" but it is "5 meters."

5) The abbreviations (e.g. "kg," "mL," "mm") are *never* made plural. 100 kg is written as "100 kg" and not "100 kgs."

6) A space is always used between the number and the metric abbreviation. For example, "5 kg," "3250 mL," or "0.5 m." This also applies to temperature (e.g. "37 °C," "98.6 °F").

7) Spaces and hyphens are never used between prefixes (e.g. "kilo," "milli") and the base word ("meter," "gram," "liter"), or between the letters of the metric abbreviation (e.g. it is always "kg" not "k g"). When spelled out, it is "milliliter", not "milli-liter" or "milli liter."

8) When a metric unit is used as a noun modifier (e.g. "2-liter bottle", which describes what kind of bottle), the metric unit is written out. Thus it is a "100-meter dash," not a "100-m dash." A hyphen is not required to be written between the numerical value and the metric unit, but either form, with or without the hyphen, is acceptable (e.g. "5 kilometer walk" or "5-kilometer walk").

9) Do not use a period after a metric abbreviation unless the abbreviation occurs at the end of a sentence (e.g. "kg" not "kg.").

10) In all numbers less than 1, the zero is always put in the space before the decimal (in the "ones" space). It is "0.5 kg" not ".5 kg."

11) When speaking about metric units, the first syllable of the prefix (e.g. "kilo," "milli," "centi") is accented, not the second syllable. Kilometer is correctly pronounced "KILL-oh-mee-ter," not "kill-OM-eh-ter."

force gravity exerts on the animal's mass to pull it towards the center of the earth. In clinics, both words are used, such when referring to the animal's *weight* or stating the *mass* of the drug that was injected into the patient. In this book, these two terms will be used in the context of how they are most commonly spoken in clinical practice.

The metric unit of mass (or weight), such as the weight of a drug in a dose or the weight of the patient, is expressed using the metric base unit *gram* with the appropriate prefix. The most commonly used units for mass are kilogram, gram, milligram, microgram, and nanogram. Notice that kilograms are 10^3 times (1000×) greater than grams, and milligrams are 10^{-3} times (0.001×) smaller than grams. Micrograms are an additional 10^{-3} (0.001×) smaller than milligrams, and nanograms are an additional 10^{-3} smaller than micrograms. Therefore, the major metric units of mass commonly used by veterinary professionals are conveniently spaced at intervals of 1000. Another way of saying this is that by moving the decimal point on a number three spaces to the right or left, allows easy conversion from one metric unit value to another.

Note that some older textbooks and publications may use "Gm" as the abbreviation for gram. This older expression is one of several that were in use prior to when the abbreviations for the metric system were standardized in 1960. The older "Gm" abbreviation for grams was used to differentiate grams from the apothecary measurement of mass called grains (gr). Today, the lowercase letter "g" represents the unit of gram and the "gr" is used for grains.

In order to convert between the metric units for mass, there are certain conversions that the veterinary professional must either memorize or mathematically conceptualize. These are shown below. With these

Table 6.3 How to make common metric mass conversions

Convert from	To	Multiply original by	Or move decimal	Example
grams (g)	kilograms (kg)	0.001	3 spaces to the left	5 g = 0.005 kg
grams (g)	milligrams (mg)	1000	3 spaces to the right	8 g = 8000 mg
grams (g)	micrograms (mcg)	1000 000 or 10^6	6 spaces to the right	4 g = 4000 000 mcg
kilograms (kg)	grams (g)	1000	3 spaces to the right	7 kg = 7000 g
kilograms (kg)	milligrams (mg)	1000 000 or 10^6	6 spaces to the right	3 kg = 3000 000 mg
milligrams (mg)	grams (g)	0.001	3 spaces to the left	2 mg = 0.002 g
milligrams (mg)	micrograms (mcg)	1000	3 spaces to the right	6 mg = 6000 mcg

commonly used units, it is a matter of moving the decimal point three places right or left depending upon whether the resulting number value is greater or less than the original value. Examples of how to make the conversions are shown in Table 6.3.

A common error is to move the decimal point in the wrong direction. Therefore, it is important to conceptualize the relative sizes one metric unit has to another. An easy way to do this is to imagine a balance scale or a teeter-totter with the amount of one metric unit on one side, and the equivalent amount of another metric unit on the other. For example, in conceptualizing a gram and kilogram relationship, start with a gram and realize that it is very small compared to a kilogram. Therefore, only a very small fraction of a kilogram is going to balance the other side of the scale or teeter-totter against the single gram on the other side. 5 g would then be equivalent to 0.005 kg, which is a very small fraction of one total kilogram. At the same time, 1 g is far larger than a milligram, so an equivalent number of milligrams needed to balance the 1 g would be huge. As an example, 2 g is the same as 2000 mg.

By stepping back and looking at the answer itself relative to the size of the patient, errors in moving the decimal point can be often be identified. For example, giving 4000 mL (4 L) of a liquid drug by IM injection to a 5 pound Chihuahua intuitively does not make sense. Therefore, take the time to evaluate the answer in each dose calculation for common sense. By practicing conversions repeatedly, the veterinary technician will develop an instinctive understanding of the relative size of an answer when making conversions between different metric units, thus reducing the chances of errors.

6.3 Metric Units of Volume

The metric units of volume use the base unit of *liter*. The most common metric units of volume are liter (L), milliliter (1 mL equals 0.001 L), and microliter (1 mcL is the same as 1 μL and equals 0.000 001 L). Other metric prefixes may be attached to the base unit liter, but the relationships to the base unit liter is identical to the relationships use for the base unit grams described in Section 6.2.

Another unit of volume commonly used in syringe volumes is the "cc" or "cubic centimeter." Although a centimeter is a unit of length, the volume described by a "cc" is a 1 cm × 1 cm × 1 cm cube and is equivalent in volume to 1 mL. Therefore, "cc" and "mL" are considered equivalent units (Figure 6.1).

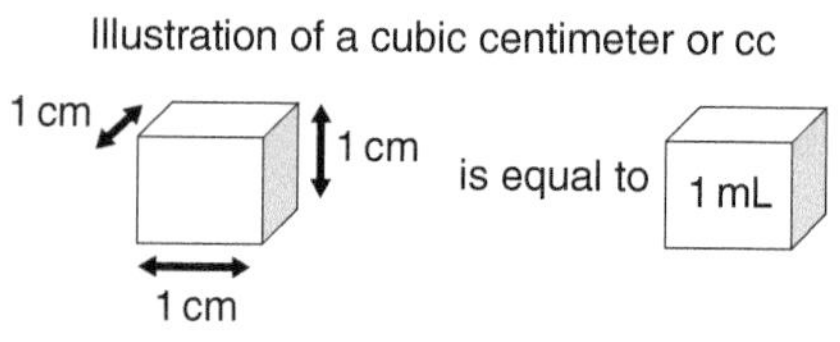

Illustration of a cubic centimeter or cc

1 cm, 1 cm, 1 cm is equal to 1 mL

Figure 6.1 1 cubic centimeter ("cc") is equivalent to 1 mL

Table 6.4 Conversions commonly used in metric volume calculations

Convert from	To	Multiply original by	Or move decimal	Example
milliliters (mL)	liter (L)	0.001	3 spaces to the left	5 mL = 0.005 L
milliliters (mL)	microliter (mcL or μL)	1000	3 spaces to the right	8 mL = 8000 μL
milliliters (mL)	cubic centimeter (cc)	1	don't move	4 mL = 4 cc
microliters (μL)	milliliters (mL)	0.001	3 spaces to the left	2 μL = 0.002 mL
liters (L)	cubic centimeter (cc)	1000	3 spaces to the right	7 L = 7000 cc
liters (L)	microliter (mcL or μL)	1000 000 or 10^6	6 spaces to the right	9 L = 9000 000 mcL

Notice that the abbreviation for liter is "L" and not a lowercase letter "l". As you can tell by the text in this book, the lowercase "l" looks remarkably like the number "1" and the capital "I". Therefore, to avoid confusion, the abbreviations for all liter measurements are written with a capitalized "L" (e.g. mL, mcL).

The commonly used conversions of metric volume are shown in Table 6.4 and should be memorized so the veterinary technician can make quick and accurate calculations of liquid doses or intravenous fluid administration.

6.4 Metric Units of Length

The basic unit of length in the metric system is the *meter*. While the meter is commonly used in Europe and Canada, in the United States the more commonly used measurement is the yard (36 in.). To conceptualize how long a meter (39.37 in.) is, suffice it to say that it is slightly longer than the "yard" (Figure 6.2).

The relationship between the base unit meter and other metric lengths is the same as for the metric units of volume and weight. The most commonly used units of metric length in veterinary medicine are meter (m), kilometer (1 km equals 1000 m), centimeter (1 cm equals 0.01 m), millimeter (1 mm equals 0.001 m), and micrometer (1 mcm is the same as 1 μm and equals 0.000 001 m). Although micrometer (or "micrometre", as spelled outside of the USA) is the official term for the metric length of 10^{-6} m, as decreed by the International System of Units in 1967, the term "micron" and the Greek symbol mu (μ) are still widely used in literature to denote the micrometer (mcm) length.

To conceptualize the length of a centimeter, an average person's thumbnail is approximately 2 cm across from side to side. The veterinary technician will see micrometers (mcm or μm) used frequently in veterinary texts or literature to describe the length of cells or organisms viewed under a microscope. To conceptualize how small this length is, a micron or micrometer is equal to 0.000 039 in., which would be roughly equivalent to two inches compared to a mile.

Figure 6.2 Comparison of 1 m to 1 yard (36 in)

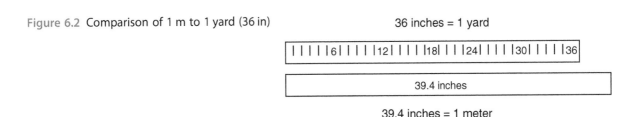

Table 6.5 Conversions commonly used in metric linear calculations

Convert from	To	Multiply original by	Or move decimal	Example
meter (m)	kilometer (km)	0.001	3 spaces to the left	5 m = 0.005 km
meter (m)	centimeter (cm)	100	2 spaces to the right	3 m = 300 cm
meter (m)	millimeter (mm)	1000	3 spaces to the right	8 m = 8000 mm
meter (m)	micrometer (mcm or μm)	1000 000 or 10^6	6 spaces to the right	9 m = 9000 000 μm
meter (m)	micron (μ)	1000 000 or 10^6	6 spaces to the right	7 m = 7000 000 μ
centimeter (cm)	millimeter (mm)	10	1 space to the right	2 cm = 20 mm
millimeter (mm)	centimeter (cm)	0.1	1 space to the left	6 mm = 0.6 cm
centimeter (cm)	meter (m)	0.01	2 spaces to the left	4 cm = 0.04 m

The veterinary technician should be able to make the following linear conversions shown in Table 6.5 without performing a calculation.

6.5 Metric Units of Concentration and Density

Metric units are combined to describe the density of an object or the concentration of a solute in a solution, such as the amount of drug that is dissolved in an amount of liquid medium. Concentrations of solutions are most commonly expressed as a unit of mass within a unit of volume. Table 6.6 shows examples of concentrations and how they might be used in veterinary medicine.

In large animal medicine and nutrition, concentrations may be expressed as a unit of mass per another unit of mass. The mass-per-mass concentration is most commonly used to describe the concentration of feed additives per unit of feed. These are sometimes also seen in describing the amount of a biologically produced toxin contained in a unit of feed. Examples are shown in Table 6.7.

Familiarity with metric units and frequent practice in converting between all metric units will greatly improve both the efficiency of calculating doses and the accuracy of those calculations.

Table 6.6 Examples of concentrations

25 mg/cc	25 mg of dexamethasone drug in each cc of liquid alcohol medium
10 g/L	10 g of disinfectant added to each liter of water
0.05 kg/100 mL	0.05 kg or 50 g of antibiotic added to each 100 mL of IV fluids

Table 6.7 Examples of how concentrations might be used to describe the mass of poison or drug per unit of feed

100 g/kg	100 g of sulfa antibiotic per kilogram of poultry feed
3 mg/100 g	3 mg of antiparasitic drug per 100 g of laboratory mice pellets
0.5 ng/kg	0.5 nanograms of coumarin toxin per kilogram of silage

6.6   Nonmetric Units: Household, Apothecary, and Avoirdupois Units

Before the metric system was developed, units of measurement were based upon common utensils (teaspoon, cup, etc.) or readily accessible measuring units (foot, rod, grain of wheat, etc.). The *apothecary measurement system* was adopted by physicians and those that compounded medications from herbs and other natural sources as a means for measuring components for creating early medications. This system only measured volume and weight and did not have a measurement for length. The *minim* was the basic unit of liquid volume and was about equivalent to one drop of water, while the *grain* was a measurement of solid weight and was about equivalent to one grain of wheat. Other measurements included fluidrams and drams. Although the apothecary system has largely been phased out from common use in veterinary medicine, vestiges of it still occasionally appear.

The *avoirdupois system* is also an older system and is the system associated with units of weight such as ounces and pounds. Some of these units are still commonly used in veterinary medicine (*grains, pounds, and ounces*), but most units have been replaced by the metric system units. Some units may be found in both the avoirdupois system and the apothecary system, but they often have different values. For example, the apothecary system "pound" equals 12 oz, but the avoirdupois "pound" is 16 oz. ("oz" is the abbreviation of "ounce".)

The *household measurement system* was actually an informal part of the avoirdupois system, but still persists today and is found in measurements used in cooking and to describe volumes of over-the-counter (OTC) consumer preparations in the USA today. Common household measurements include *drops* (gtt), *teaspoon* (tsp), *tablespoon* (Tbsp), *fluid ounce* (fl oz), *cups* (c), *pint* (pt), *quart* (qt), and *gallon* (gal).

Although "medical drops" have an official drop-to-mL conversion of 1 drop = 0.05 mL (20 drips = 1 mL), the more common use of drop-to-mL conversion occurs when calculating intravenous fluid rates where X number of drops observed in the drip chamber of the IV tubing apparatus equals 1 mL. However, this drop-to-mL conversion varies between brands or types of drip chambers, and depending upon the particular drip chamber the conversion may be calibrated such that 1 mL of liquid is delivered in 10 drips, 15 drips, 20 drips, or 60 drips. Each IV tubing set indicates on its packaging the calibration for the drip chamber incorporated into the IV set. Thus, the scientific conversion of 1 drip to 0.05 mL (20 drips per mL) does not always apply when converting the number of drips observed in an IV apparatus drip chamber to its equivalent mL volume.

The non-metric units in Table 6.8 constitute the most commonly used in veterinary medicine and should be committed to memory. Their abbreviations and metric equivalents are also listed in Table 6.8.

The number of milliliters found in cups, pints, and quarts makes it easy to have half, third, and quarter fractions of these units that are still expressed in a whole number. For example, a half cup = 120 mL, a third cup = 80 mL, and a quarter cup = 60 mL. Even though these household measurement volumes are used more in cooking than medical situations, the easy conversion between these household measurements and metric measurements makes for easy translation of recipes or formulas expressed as milliliters into cups or quarts, and vice versa.

Table 6.8 Common conversions between metric and non-metric units

Weight				
2.2 pound	=	2.2 lb	=	1 kg
1 grain	=	1 gr	=	60 or ~65 mg
Volume				
1 teaspoon	=	1 t or tsp	=	5 mL
1 tablespoon	=	1 T or Tbsp	=	15 mL
1 fluid ounce	=	1 fl oz	=	30 mL
1 cup	=	1 c	=	240 mL
1 pint	=	1 pt	=	480 mL
1 quart	=	1 qt	=	960 mL
1 gal	=	1 gal	=	3.84 L

Note that the units of "pint," "quart," and "gallon" represent different volumes in Canada and the United Kingdom and go under the designation of "imperial gallon," "imperial quart," or "imperial pint" (although in those countries the "imperial" part of the description may be assumed and therefore dropped). While the *ratio* of pint to quart and gallon remains the same in both US and imperial versions (1 gal equals 4 quarts equals 8 pints), the actual volume represented is different, with 1 imperial gallon being equivalent to 1.2 US gallons (4.8 US quarts or 9.6 US pints). For purposes of this text, these household measurements will be defined according to the standards in the USA, but it is important to remember that different volumes are used outside of the USA.

Another important distinction is between an "ounce" (oz) and "fluid ounce" (fl oz). Often when spoken or written, the descriptor "fluid" is left off and it is up to the reader to determine if the ounce in question is a volume (fluid ounce) or a mass (ounce). A fluid ounce is defined for purposes of food and medication in the USA as 30 mL and an ounce is 1/16th of a pound (as there are 16 oz of mass in one pound). As would be expected, the imperial fluid ounce is a different volume from the fluid ounce used in the USA. Because the value assigned to "ounce" can be different depending upon the country in which it is used, as a general rule the use of "ounce" in medical calculations or dispensing information should be avoided.

Note that the measurement for grain is officially listed by the International System of Units as being equivalent to 64.798 91 mg. Although generally discouraged, the apothecary grain measurement is still used by some manufacturers of older medications such as aspirin and phenobarbital as either approximately 65 mg (aspirin) or 60 mg (phenobarbital) being equivalent to 1 grain. For example, "5 gr" can be found listed as "300 mg of phenobarbital" or "325 mg of aspirin". In most cases, when medication is listed by grains, the metric equivalent is also listed on the bottle or container. For purposes of this text, we will use the 60 mg equals 1 grain conversion.

The use of the single-letter abbreviations for tablespoon ("T") and teaspoon ("t") should be avoided in handwritten instructions or records because of the ease with which a poorly handwritten lowercase "t" can resemble an upper case "T," and vice versa. Because it takes 3 teaspoons to equal the volume of 1 tablespoon, there is a potential for a significant miscalculation of dose if the unit abbreviation for teaspoon is misread as the abbreviation for tablespoon. Although the abbreviation for tablespoon is occasionally listed in some sources as "tbsp", it should always be written with the uppercase "T" as "Tbsp." A tablespoon (Tbsp) is equivalent to 15 mL and a teaspoon (tsp) is equivalent to 5 mL for food or medication. It is important to note that an actual teaspoon utensil, such as those you will have in your home, has no standard volume and can vary from 2.5 mL to 6 mL volume. Thus, if using the teaspoon or tablespoon volume when dispensing medication, the client or pet owner should also be given a syringe or calibrated dispensing instrument to assure accurate dosing of the medication.

Table 6.9 Common household measurements and their equivalents (US measurements)

1 Tbsp	=	3 tsp				
1 oz	=	2 Tbsp				
1 c	=	8 oz				
1 pt	=	2 c	=	16 oz		
1 qt	=	2 pt	=	4 c	=	32 oz
1 gal	=	4 qt	=	8 pt		

Household measurements are often used in daily living and therefore how a pint relates to an equivalent quart or a gallon may already be known. Thus, memorizing one conversion from a household to its equivalent metric measurement can provide a starting point from where other conversions can be extrapolated. For example, if the conversion of 1 Tbsp to the equivalent 15 mL is memorized, and the information in the Table 6.9 is remembered, the other metric equivalents for household measurements can be determined.

Because 1 Tbsp is equivalent to 15 mL and that there are 2 Tbsp in an ounce, 1 oz must equal 30 mL (2 × 15 mL). Taking the extrapolation further, 1 c (cup) must equal 240 mL (2 × 8 × 15 mL) and 1 pt (pint) must equal 480 mL (2 × 8 × 2 × 15 mL). Because dosages are typically listed in metric units, but dispensing drug formulations or other compounds used in veterinary medicine are sometimes listed as household volumes, the veterinary professional needs to be able to convert between household units and the metric system.

6.7 Conversion between Quantities of Volume and Mass: Special Cases

The final commonly used conversion we need to look at approximates the conversion of a liquid volume to mass (weight) and is embodied by the phrases: "A pint's a pound, the world around" and "A liter of water weighs 1 kilogram." Although both phrases provide a workable estimation for *water* volume-to-weight conversions (a US pint of water weighs 1.043 75 pounds; a liter of water does weigh 1 kg), the rules do not apply to fluids with densities different from water (e.g. oil, emulsions, suspensions, saturated solutions). The "1 liter equals 1 kg" conversion is commonly used to estimate the amount of IV fluid replacement needed in an animal based upon the estimated percent dehydration (based upon clinical signs) and the patient's body weight (in kilograms). Thus, a 10 kg patient with signs of 5% dehydration is presumed to have lost 0.5 kg of weight of body water (5% × 10 kg equals 0.05 × 10 kg equals 0.5 kg) and therefore needs 0.5 L (500 mL) of fluid to replace what has been lost. The pint to pound conversion and the other conversions shown in Table 6.10 are often used to approximate the weight of a liquid within container of a known volume (e.g. 10 gal aquarium equals 40 quarts equals 80 pints equals 80 lbs of weight). It is important to remember that a US pint is different from the imperial pint in that a US pint is 16 fluid ounces while the imperial pint is larger at 20 fluid ounces. This means that the "pint to pound" conversion wouldn't be as accurate for the imperial volumes.

Table 6.10 Conversion of household measurement of water volume to approximate weight

"A pint's a pound the world around"
1 pint (pt) = 1 pound (lb)
16 fluid ounces = 1 pound (lb)
1 quart = 2 pounds (lb)
1 gallon = 8 pounds (lb)

6.8 Converting Between Units: The Proportion and Cancel-Out Methods

Because medications, compounds, and delivery systems (e.g. syringes, bags of intravenous fluids) may come in metric or nonmetric units of measurement, the key equivalents should be memorized in order to facilitate making the conversions. We will focus here on the conversions most commonly used in veterinary medicine.

The most commonly used conversion, and one often confused during conversion from one system to another, is the conversion between kilogram and pounds. A simple way to remember whether the "number" gets larger or smaller when converting from pounds to kilograms and vice versa, is to determine your own weight in both pounds and kilograms. Because 2.2 lb equals only 1 kg, a person would become much "slimmer" when their body weight is converted from pounds to kilograms. For example, a 220 lb football linebacker becomes a 100 kg "weakling" when his weight is converted to the metric system. Another rhyming phrase used to help remember this is: "If you start with pound, your kilograms go down."

It is important to keep this relationship in mind so that *every* pound-to-kilogram conversion answer is mentally checked to make sure the increase or decrease in numerical value makes sense. Try these two examples and decide which of the alternatives is the correct answer.

> Does a 40 lb dog weigh 18.2 kg or 88 kg?
> Does a 20 kg dog weighs 9.1 lb or 44 lb?

The "40 lb dog" converts to a smaller number in kilograms (18.2 kg) while a "20 kg dog" weighs 44 lbs.

Conversion between most metric units is performed simply by mentally moving the decimal point the number of positions as described in Sections 6.2, 6.3, and 6.4. However, when converting from nonmetric units to metric units (or vice versa), the conversions are typically not so easily performed. Therefore, it is important to set up a system by which any conversion can be made in a consistently accurate and reliable manner. By choosing one method for calculating conversions that makes sense and by using the same method all the time, consistency in producing the correct answer is increased.

Two basic methods will be introduced at this point. They are often called by a variety of different names, but will be referred to in this text as the *proportion* method and the *cancel-out* method. Algebraically, they are very similar in their methodology, but they are set up slightly differently. Each is equally reliable if the rules for each method are remembered and practiced. Pick one, become very familiar with it, and use it!

6.8.1   Using the Proportion Method

The weight of a 66 lb animal needs to be converted into the equivalent kilogram weight. Three things need to be identified to correctly set up this problem:

1) the given or known value and its units (66 lb),
2) the unit of the unknown value X to which the given value is to be converted (kilogram), and
3) a "conversion factor" that describes the relationship of the given to the unknown (2.2 lb equals 1 kg).

The "conversion factor" is any equivalent equation in which the units of the given known value and the unknown units are both used. In the example above, 66 pounds are being converted to an unknown X number of kilograms, so a conversion factor that defines the relationship between pounds and kilograms is needed. In this case, the conversion factor of 1 kg equals 2.2 lb previously mentioned works nicely for this purpose, although any variation of this relationship could also be used (e.g. 10 kg equals 22 lb, 0.454 kg equals 1 lb, etc.).

In the proportion method, the problem is set up as a proportion of values on either side of an equation, using the general format shown below:

$$\frac{\text{unknown } X \text{ unit}}{\text{known value unit}} = \frac{\text{conversion factor with same units as unknown } X}{\text{conversion factor with same units as known value}}$$

For converting 66 lb animal to the unknown X kg animal the "kg" units are put into the unknown X part of the problem (in this case, the numerator on the left side of the equation) and the known "66 lb" is put into the known value unit (denominator on the left side of the equation):

$$\frac{X \text{ kg}}{\text{known value unit}} = \frac{\text{conversion factor with same units as unknown } X}{\text{conversion factor with same units as known value}}$$

$$\frac{X \text{ kg}}{66 \text{ lb}} = \frac{\text{conversion factor with same units as unknown } X}{\text{conversion factor with same units as known value}}$$

The right side of the equation contains the conversion factor which is the description of the relationship between kilograms and pounds (1 kg equals 2.2 lb). The components of the conversion factor are placed into the proportional equation so that similar units (the kilogram or pound units) are on the top and bottom for both sides of the fraction. In this case, since the "X kg" is in the numerator (top) part of the fraction on the left, the conversion on the right is set up with the "kg" unit in the numerator part of the conversion fraction.

$$\frac{X \text{ kg}}{66 \text{ lb}} = \frac{\text{conversion factor with same units as unknown } X}{\text{conversion factor with same units as known value}}$$

$$\frac{X \text{ kg}}{66 \text{ lb}} = \frac{1 \text{ kg}}{2.2 \text{ lb}}$$

The problem is now set up in the proper configuration to solve for the unknown X as described in Chapter 5. As described in Chapter 5, the unknown X must be isolated to one side of the equation and in this example this is accomplished by moving the "1/66 lb" to the right side of the equation. This is accomplished by multiplying both sides of the equation by "66 lb". Note that the units *must* be included with the numerical value. The "66 lb" in the numerator "cancels" the 66 lb in the denominator of the "X kg/66 lb" fraction. In reality, the "1/66 lb" is being multiplied by its reciprocal "66 lb" which yields the value of 1 (as described in Chapter 5).

$$\frac{X \text{ kg}}{66 \text{ lb}} = \frac{1 \text{ kg}}{2.2 \text{ lb}}$$

$$66 \text{ lb} \times \frac{X \text{ kg}}{66 \text{ lb}} = \frac{1 \text{ kg}}{2.2 \text{ lb}} \times 66 \text{ lb}$$

cancel the 66 lb: $\quad \cancel{66 \text{ lb}} \times \dfrac{X \text{ kg}}{\cancel{66 \text{ lb}}} = \dfrac{1 \text{ kg}}{2.2 \text{ lb}} \times 66 \text{ lb}$

cancel the lb: $\quad X \text{ kg} = \dfrac{1 \text{ kg}}{2.2 \cancel{\text{ lb}}} \times 66 \cancel{\text{ lb}}$

$$X \text{ kg} = \frac{1 \text{ kg} \times 66}{2.2}$$

$$X \text{ kg} = 30 \text{ kg}$$

Notice that the only unit left in the equation at the end is the "kg" and all units of "lb" have been eliminated from the equation. This principle of eliminating all of the units except for the unit associated with the unknown X is key to knowing that the problem has been correctly set up. Once the unknown X has been isolated in the problem above, the unit "lb" in the numerator with "66 lb" can be canceled by the "lb" unit in the denominator with "2.2 lb", leaving only the unit for "kg" on the right side of the equation which matches the "kg" unit for the unknown X.

The problem is set up correctly because when the calculation is finished the answer on the right side will be expressed as "kg," which is the same unit as the unknown X. Had the problem not been set up correctly, the "lb" units would not have canceled each other out and the right-side calculated answer would have been inappropriately expressed in some combination of "lb" and "kg" units.

The answer for this proportional method calculation is checked by plugging the 30 kg solution into the original equation to see if the same numerical value is obtained on either side of the equal sign.

$$\frac{X \text{ kg}}{66 \text{ lb}} = \frac{1 \text{ kg}}{2.2 \text{ lb}}$$

$$\frac{30\,kg}{66\,lb} = \frac{1\,kg}{2.2\,lb}$$

$$\frac{0.454\,kg}{lb} = \frac{0.454\,kg}{lb}$$

Because both sides of the equations have the same value, the answer of 30 kg for X is correct!

Here is an example of using the proportional method to convert from one metric unit (g) to another (kg):

How many kilograms are in a 340 g bottle?

$$\frac{unknown\,X\,unit}{known\,value\,unit} = \frac{conversion\,factor\,with\,same\,units\,as\,unknown\,X}{conversion\,factor\,with\,same\,units\,as\,known\,value}$$

$$\frac{X\,kg}{340\,g} = \frac{conversion\,factor\,with\,same\,units\,as\,unknown\,X}{conversion\,factor\,with\,same\,units\,as\,known\,value}$$

$$\frac{X\,kg}{340\,g} = \frac{1\,kg}{1000\,g}$$

$$340\,g \times \frac{X\,kg}{340\,g} = \frac{1\,kg}{1000\,g} \times 340\,g$$

$$\cancel{340\,g} \times \frac{X\,kg}{\cancel{340\,g}} = \frac{1\,kg}{1000\,g} \times 340\,g$$

$$X\,kg = \frac{1\,kg}{1000\,g} \times 340\,g$$

$$X\,kg = \frac{1\,kg}{1000\,\cancel{g}} \times 340\,\cancel{g}$$

$$X\,kg = \frac{1\,kg}{1000} \times 340$$

$$X\,kg = \frac{340\,kg}{1000}$$

$$X\,kg = 0.34\,kg$$

The problem was set up correctly because the unit of the answer (kg) was the same as the unit of the unknown X (kg), and all other units had been canceled out or eliminated. Check the answer by plugging 0.34 back into the original equation. Note that when checking the answer, the units can be ignored. The focus is just on the numerical value since the appropriate canceling of units was checked by having the unit on the right side of the equation the same as the unit needed for the unknown X in the original calculation above.

$$\frac{X\,kg}{340\,g} = \frac{1\,kg}{1000\,g}$$

$$\frac{0.34}{340} = \frac{1}{1000}$$

$$0.001 = 0.001$$

6.8.2 Using the Cancel-out Method

This method is sometimes called the "factor-label method," "unit conversion," or "dimensional analysis." By calling it the "cancel-out" method, we are describing how this method works and how it is set up. No matter what name is used, the key principle of this method requires setting up a multiplication problem so that all the units (milligram, kilogram, milliliter, etc.) cancel each other out leaving only the unit used for the unknown X.

To set up a problem in the cancel-out method, the unknown is put on one side of the equation, and then the known value and conversion factors are arranged into a multiplication problem on the other side of the equation. In arranging the multiplication problem, all of the units are set up so that a unit in the numerator (top number in a fraction) "cancels" with the identical unit in the denominator (the bottom number), as was described in the proportional method (Section 6.8.1). If the problem has been set up properly, all of the units but one will cancel out, leaving only the unit used for the unknown X in the numerator position. Once this problem is properly arranged the problem is multiplied to calculate the answer. Here is the general equation:

$$\text{unknown } X \text{ unit} = \text{known value unit} \times \frac{\text{conversion factor with same units as unknown } X}{\text{conversion factor with same units as known value}}$$

This can be demonstrated using as an example the same problem used in the proportion method. "How many kilograms is a 66 lb animal?" In that problem, the unknown X was expressed in kilograms, a known value of 66 was given in pounds (lb), and a conversion factor of 2.2 lb equals 1 kg was used. To start, the unknown X and its unit are placed on one side of the equal sign:

$$X \text{ kg} =$$

On the other side of the equation, the known value (66 lb) and the conversion factor (2.2 lb = 1 kg) are arranged so that the given known units (lb) are in the numerator and denominator, thus canceling each other out, leaving only the unknown X unit (kg) above the line in the numerator position.

$$X \text{ kg} = 66 \text{ lb} \times \frac{1 \text{ kg}}{2.2 \text{ lb}}$$

$$X \text{ kg} = 66 \cancel{\text{lb}} \times \frac{1 \text{ kg}}{2.2 \cancel{\text{lb}}}$$

$$X \text{ kg} = 66 \times \frac{1 \text{ kg}}{2.2}$$

When the calculation is performed, the unit in the answer on the right side of the equation matches the unit of the unknown X (kg).

$$X \text{ kg} = \frac{66 \text{ kg}}{2.2}$$

$$X \text{ kg} = 30 \text{ kg}$$

An advantage of the cancel-out method is that there is only *one* way to *correctly* set up the right side of the equation so that the pound units cancel and that leaves only the kilogram unit above the line (in the numerator).

If the equation had been improperly set up (as shown below) and the answer multiplied through, the resulting units would have looked rather peculiar:

$$X\,kg = 66\,lb \times \frac{2.2\,lb}{1\,kg}$$

$$X\,kg = \frac{145.2\,lb^2}{kg}$$

The "lb^2" unit in the answer results from multiplying "66 lb" and "2.2 lb", giving the answer as "square pounds" ("lb^2") over kilograms which renders the answer useless because of the units.

The other advantage of the cancel-out method is the ability to set up rather complex problems and to know that the problem is correctly arranged based on the ability to cancel out all units except the unit in the answer. For example, a dog needed 0.2 g of a drug, but the medication to be administered was in a liquid form and the concentration on the label was in milligrams and listed as 100 mg/mL. In this problem the dose of 0.2 g has to be converted into the milligrams of drug needed from the bottle. But ultimately the milligrams of drugs needs to be translated into a number of milliliters (mL) of liquid to be withdrawn from the bottle. In this case, the unknown *X* for the final answer would be the number of mL needed for the dog, the known value would be the dog's dose of 0.2 g, and the two conversion factors would be the conversion from grams to milligrams (1 g = 1000 mg) and the conversion of mg to mL listed as the drug concentration on the bottle's label. 100 mg/mL means that there is 100 mg drug in every mL of liquid. The unknown *X* (mL) is put on one side of the equation, and the known and conversion factors are put on the other side. Here is a first attempt at this:

$$X\,mL = 0.2\,g \times \frac{1\,g}{1000\,mg} \times \frac{100\,mg}{1\,mL}$$

However, this set up violates a couple of rules needed to correctly set up this problem. First, the answer unit (mL) is not in the numerator (top part) of the fraction on the right side of this equation. That needs to be corrected first. Here is a second attempt:

$$X\,mL = 0.2\,g \times \frac{1\,g}{1000\,mg} \times \frac{1\,mL}{100\,mg}$$

But in this configuration the "mg" units and the "g" units cannot cancel out because the units are not present in both the numerator and denominator. Both the "mg" are in the denominator and both the "g" are in the numerator. By flipping the 1 g/1000 mg conversion factor, the mg and g units can be canceled out. Here is the third, and final, attempt:

$$X\,mL = 0.2\,g \times \frac{1000\,mg}{1\,g} \times \frac{1\,mL}{100\,mg}$$

Looking at the right side of the equation, the "mg" units can now cancel with each other (because one is in the numerator and one is in the denominator) and the "g" units can also cancel. This will leave only the "mL" unit on top, which is the correct position for the unit needed for the unknown *X*.

$$X\,\text{mL} = 0.2\,\cancel{g} \times \frac{1000\,\text{mg}}{1\,\cancel{g}} \times \frac{1\,\text{mL}}{100\,\text{mg}}$$

$$X\,\text{mL} = 0.2 \times \frac{1000\,\cancel{\text{mg}}}{1} \times \frac{1\,\text{mL}}{100\,\cancel{\text{mg}}}$$

$$X\,\text{mL} = 0.2 \times \frac{1000}{1} \times \frac{1\,\text{mL}}{100}$$

$$X\,\text{mL} = \frac{0.2 \times 1000 \times 1\,\text{mL}}{1 \times 100}$$

$$X\,\text{mL} = \frac{200\,\text{mL}}{100}$$

$$X\,\text{mL} = 2\,\text{mL}$$

The 0.2 g of drug needed for this dog would be administered in 2 mL of liquid medication at the concentration of 100 mg of drug per 1 mL of liquid medication. By setting up all of the conversion factors in a manner that all units canceled except for the unit needed for the answer, we know that the problem was correctly arranged to find the correct answer.

In order to be consistently correct in doing dosage calculations, it is important to pick one method (proportion or cancel-out) that works best for you and to practice it repeatedly so that you will become very familiar with how the problem needs to be set up to produce the correct answer.

6.9   Estimating the Answer: Does Your Answer Make Sense?

As experience is gained calculating doses for a particular drug over and over again, an appreciation is formed for approximately how much of the drug will be needed for a 10, 20, or 50 lb animal. Thus, if a mistake in calculating the dose is made, there is an instinctive feeling that the calculated answer "doesn't look right." Although this developed perspective should never replace double checking or triple checking a calculated dose, it can be useful as an additional safety check. This skill of estimating an expected general range of acceptable answers to a dosing calculation can be developed more quickly by practicing estimating the approximate answer to basic dosing exercises without using a calculator.

People already make estimations in other aspects of life, from guessing the total of the grocery bill to stay within the budget, or estimating the cost of gasoline needed to fill a car's gas tank. In a veterinary applied example, if the drug dose for a 10 lb dog is known, it should be easy to quickly estimate the dose for a 20 lb dog without using a calculator as it is almost intuitive to know that a 20 lb dog gets twice the dose as the 10 lb dog.

Estimating changes that result in half or double amounts is pretty easy. Estimating one-quarter (25%) or three-quarter (75%) dose changes uses the same ideas but repeats the steps. For example, if an 80 lb dog requires 100 mg, how much does a 20 lb dog need? The difference is that 20 lb is one-quarter of the 80 lb weight, so either the original dose can be divided mentally by four to give one-quarter of the dose (100 mg becomes 25 mg), or you can halve the original dose (100 mg becomes 50 mg) and then halve it again (50 mg becomes 25 mg) because half of one-half is equal to one-quarter.

Practice making these estimations without a calculator to determine the correct dose.

- Given that a 5 lb cat needs 2 cc, how many cubic centimeters should a 10 lb cat get?
- Given that a 40 lb dog received 20 mg, how much should a 20 lb dog receive?
- Given that a 600 kg animal needs 200 mg of drug, how much does a 150 kg animal need?
- Given that the dose for a 3 lb dog is 10 g, what is the dose for a 12 lb dog?
- A 25 g rat needs 0.2 cc of a drug. How much does an 100 g rat need?
- If an 8 lb cat received 0.1 g of drug, how much did a 2 lb cat receive?

The answers would be 4 cc, 10 mg, 50 mg, 40 g, 0.8 cc, and 0.025 g (*not* 0.25 g).

These estimations of ratios working in doubles and fourths are fairly simple. Unfortunately, most calculations are not this simple so there are some other tricks that can be done to estimate a relative size of a quantity wanted for an answer. Sometimes a larger number (like "423") can be temporarily reduced and rounded to a single digit, keeping in mind how many places the decimal point was moved in making the simplification, then the calculation can be carried out.

For example, a swine producer's 423 lb boar stud needs medication at 5 mg/lb. It is far easier to multiply "4 × 5" than "423 × 5," so reduce and round "423" to "4", keeping in mind this is a reduction of 100× (or moving the decimal point two places). "4 × 5" gives 20 and since the 423 was reduced by 100× (two decimal places), the two decimal places are added back to the "20" to give 2000 for an estimate of the dose. The actual calculated dose is 2115 and that is relatively close to the 2000 derived as an estimate.

So the steps in estimating a dose are:

1) Round numbers in the problem to the nearest whole number, tens, hundreds, thousands, etc.
2) "Take away" the extra zeroes or move the decimal point. Make sure you remember how many zeroes there were or how many decimal places were moved!
3) Perform the simplified equation in your head.
4) "Add" the zeroes back to the answer or move the decimal to give your final estimate.

Use these steps for estimating this dose: a 280 lb cow needs a dose of 8 mg/lb.

1) The 280 can be rounded to 300 (nearest hundreds).
2) The two zeros can be removed to give a simple "3."
3) The simplified estimate calculation is then performed mentally: 3 × 8 = 24.
4) Add the two zeroes back to the answer to give the estimate: 24 becomes 2400 for the estimate.

The actual dose for this cow is 2240 mg, which is pretty close to the mental estimate. Again, the idea is that the estimate can be performed in a matter of seconds mentally and then compared to the actual calculated answer to ensure a large error in calculation was not accidentally made.

Practice making these estimations without a calculator to determine the correct dose.

- 32 lb dog needing 5 mg/lb
- 432 lb pony needing 8 mg/lb
- 9.7 lb cat needing 15 mg/lb
- 279 kg calf needing 4 mg/kg

The estimates should have come out to 150 mg (actual is 160 mg), 3200 mg (actual is 3456 mg), 150 mg (actual is 145.5 mg), and 1200 mg (actual is 1116 mg).

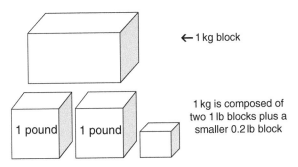

Figure 6.3 Comparison of 2.2 pounds to 1 kg

One of the hardest things for those learning to make these body weight conversions between pounds and kilograms to remember is whether the conversion is 2.2 lb = 1 kg or if it is the other way around. It can help to visualize the kilogram block shown in Figure 6.3 and how it is composed of two 1 lb blocks plus a smaller 0.2 lb block. In order to balance the relatively "big" kilogram block on a scale or teeter-tooter opposite of the units of pounds, more than one "lb" block would have to be used. Thus, it takes 2.2 pounds (lb) to equal 1 kilogram (kg).

For estimating this conversion from pounds to kilograms (2.2 pounds = 1 kg), it's easy to round the "2.2" to "2" to perform the conversion calculation to pounds.

For example, a 66 pound dog needs a drug whose dose is listed as "mg/kg." The "66 pounds" needs to be converted to the equivalent kilograms before the dose calculation can be performed. This conversion would require dividing 66 by 2.2. If written out, this would appear as shown below:

$$66\,\text{lb} \times \frac{\text{kg}}{2.2\,\text{lb}} = X\,\text{kg}$$

Because this exercise is a mental estimation of the eventual answer, the "2.2" can be replaced by "2," meaning the dog's weight in pounds is divided by 2 to give an approximation of the kilogram equivalent.

$$\text{estimate by}: 66\,\text{lb} \times \frac{\text{kg}}{2\,\text{lb}}$$

$$\text{lb units cancel out, leaving kg on top}: \frac{66\,\text{kg}}{2}$$

$$\frac{66\,\text{kg}}{2} = 33\,\text{kg}$$

Thus, to estimate the conversion from pounds to kilograms, the pound weight can be divided by 2. For the problem above, when the actual pound-to-kilogram calculation is done the answer is 30 kg, which is close to the 33 kg arrived doing the quick estimate.

To estimate the conversion the other way (kilograms to pounds), the kilogram "number" would have to be *multiplied* by 2. Remember to visualize the equivalent number of "blocks" of pounds needed to balance 1 kg in Figure 6.3.

Practice making these pound to kilogram estimations, without a calculator:

- 4.4 lb = ??? kg
- 20 lb = ??? kg
- 880 lb = ??? kg
- 1240 lb = ??? kg

The estimates should be 2.2 kg (actual is 2 kg), 10 kg (actual is 9.01 kg), 440 kg (actual is 400 kg), and 620 kg (actual is 563.6363 kg).

Practice making these kilogram to pound estimations, without a calculator:

- 10 kg = ??? lb
- 25 kg = ??? lb
- 2.2 kg = ??? lb
- 0.1 kg = ??? lb

The estimates should be 20 (actual is 22 lb), 50 (actual is 55 lb), 4.4 (actual is 4.84 lb), and 0.2 lb (actual is 0.22 lb).

6.10   Chapter 6 Practice Problems

1   Write the decimal number and the unit abbreviations that would be used for each of the following:

A) twenty kilograms
B) ten point three milliliters
C) thirty-five cubic centimeters
D) five and one-tenth milligrams
E) thirty-four and two-hundredth grams
F) twenty-six and forty-three thousandth liters
G) fifteen milligrams per kilogram
H) zero point zero one four grams per liter
I) one point two five micrometers
J) zero point five grains
K) twenty pounds
L) thirty-five teaspoons
M) five and one-half tablespoons
N) three point two five fluid ounces
O) six and one-fourth cups
P) fifteen gallons
Q) zero point five quarts

2   Make the following metric conversions:

A) 340 mg = _____ g
B) 0.325 kg = _____ g = _____ mg
C) 52 mL = _____ cc = _____ L
D) 0.0251 L = _____ mL
E) 3 km = _____ m
F) 40 cm = _____ mm = _____ m
G) 0.355 m = _____ cm = _____ mm
H) 2.5 km = _____ m
I) 0.0003 kg = _____ mg
J) 3876 mm = _____ cm = _____ m

3   Make the following conversions between metric and nonmetric units:

A) 55 lb = _____ kg
B) 4.4 lb = _____ kg
C) 20 kg = _____ lb

D) 4 tsp = _____ mL = _____ L
E) 25 Tbsp = _____ mL = _____ L
F) 90 mL = _____ tsp = _____ Tbsp
G) 90 mg = _____ gr = _____ g
H) 0.6 kg = _____ g = _____ gr = _____ lb

4 A dog with epilepsy is being treated with 1/4 gr phenobarbital every 12 hours. How many *milligrams* of phenobarbital is the patient receiving *per day*?

5 If an animal is supposed to receive 3 tsp daily of a prescribed liquid medication, and the client only has a 3 cc syringe with which to administer the drug by mouth, how many cc's of medication are going to have to be administered with each dose? How full syringes are needed to give the whole dose?

6 You have been given orders to administer medication to a cow weighing approximately 850 pounds. Unfortunately, the dose listed in your drug formulary is listed as milligrams per kilogram of body weight requiring you to convert body weight pounds to kilograms. How many kilograms does this cow weigh?

7 The concentration of a feed additive listed on a new container of powdered additives you just purchased is 100 mg of additive/kg of powder in which it is mixed. The concentration for the same type of feed additive listed on another package from another manufacturer is 0.1 kg additive/kg of powder. Are the concentrations of feed additive per kilogram of powder equivalent for these two products?

8 Mrs. Jones calls the veterinary hospital and says her dog has just consumed 15 tablets of a 1/2 gr OTC (over-the-counter) medication that spilled on the floor. The veterinarian looks up the drug and calculates what a potentially lethal dose would be for a dog the size of Mrs. Jones' pet and determines that the dog would have to consume 0.5 g of drug to produce a significant toxicosis, and 0.75 g of drug is lethal for most animals of this size. How many grams of drug did this dog ingest? Did this animal ingest a dose that will produce toxic signs or be potentially lethal?

9 The veterinarian drew up enough injectable anesthetic to safely anesthetize a 4.5 kg dog. However, the weight of the patient that will receive this anesthetic dose is 4.5 pounds, not 4.5 kg. Is this amount of anesthetic that was drawn up an overdose, an underdose, or just about right for this patient?

10 You have 35 mg of an analgesic/sedative injectable preanesthetic left in the bottle. According to the manufacturer's label dosage, 35 mg will provide analgesia and sedation for about 140 lb of animals. How many total kilograms of animal will you be able to anesthetize with the 35 mg of drug? You are going to administer the 35 mg of analgesic/sedative drug to the following animals in the order shown below. The 35 mg of drug won't be enough to sedate all of the animals. Which animal in the order below is not going to have enough drug to receive a full dose?

Patient's name	Patient's weight in kilograms
Sam	23 kg
Bert	10 kg
Lilly	16.5 kg
Zamphire	2.7 kg
Ignatz	4.3 kg
Poindexter	5.1 kg
Shubert	4.2 kg
Wussbaby	3.5 kg
Princess	6.0 kg

11   Practice estimating the answers to the following questions in your head without paper, pencil, or calculator:

    A) $23 + 19 + 43 + 58 = ???$
    B) $121 + 3522 + 889 + 39 = ???$
    C) $461 - 322 = ???$
    D) $892 - 489 = ???$
    E) $30 \times 61 = ???$
    F) $110 \times 49 = ???$
    G) $485 \div 6 = ???$

7

Understanding Drug Orders and Drug Labels

OBJECTIVES

The student will be able to:

1) identify the components of a dosage regimen either in written or in spoken form,
2) accurately use the common abbreviations for dose intervals, routes of administration, and dosage forms, and
3) read and accurately interpret a dose label and extract the information needed to calculate a dose, handle and store the medication properly, and double check that the dosage formulation is safe to use by the route of administration requested.

Some of the more common errors made in administering drugs result from misunderstood communication between the veterinarian and the veterinary technician. Drug orders may be poorly written, the drug name may be confused with another similarly spelled drug or a drug with a similar sounding name, or the volume of drug withdrawn from a vial may be inappropriate because the drug concentration in the vial is not the same as the drug concentration prescribed in the drug order. Under high-pressure, chaotic circumstances (e.g. emergency situations), the chance for dosage mistakes resulting from written or oral miscommunications increases.

To ensure patient safety, as well as the safety of the veterinary team and the animal owner, it is essential that the veterinary professional develop a strong understanding of what constitutes appropriate drug dosing orders and how to accurately write, read, and interpret such drug orders.

7.1   The Dosage Regimen

Here is an example of a correctly written dosage regimen: "15 mg given by mouth every 8 hours for 10 days." In this example, and for each correctly communicated dosage regimen, there should be four components that describe how the drug is to be administered:

1) the *dose* or the mass of drug to be given (e.g. 15 mg, 60 grains, 0.1 g)
2) the *route* by which the drug is to be given (e.g. intramuscular [IM], intravenous [IV], by mouth [PO])
3) the frequency or *dose interval* by which the drug is to be given (e.g. every 12 hours, once daily, as needed)
4) the *duration* the medication is to be given.

The duration will not be listed in the dosage regimen if the drug is only to be given one time.

Medical Mathematics and Dosage Calculations for Veterinary Technicians, Third Edition. Robert Bill.
© 2019 John Wiley & Sons, Inc. Published 2019 by John Wiley & Sons, Inc.
Companion website: www.wiley.com/go/bill/calculations

7.1.1   The Dosage Regimen: Doses and Dosages

The terms "dose" and "dosage" are often used interchangeably. However, the terms do have different meanings and different appropriate uses. The *dose* of a drug is the amount of the drug expressed as a mass of drug (e.g. milligrams, grams, grains) needed for a *specific* animal (e.g. a 30 lb dog, a 4 kg cat). The *dosage* is used as a formula to determine the individual dose for *any* animal and is typically expressed as drug mass per unit of body weight (e.g. 5 mg/kg, 10 mg/lb). For example, a reference text might list a *dosage* for Drug A as 10 mg/lb for any animal, but a specific 30 lb dog would have an administered *dose* of 300 mg of Drug A.

"Dose" and "dosage" are like "mile" and "mileage," or "acre" and "acreage." In each case the "-age" on the end refers to a "collection" of the single units. Your car travels a mile, but the accumulated collection of miles it has traveled is its mileage. An acre is one unit, and acreage is the collection of acres. The *dosage regimen* therefore is a description of how multiple individual doses are going to be used to treat an animal.

Sometimes a drug's dosage formula is expressed as a range instead of a single dosage. For example, the dosage may be listed as "1–3 mg/kg" meaning the veterinarian has the option to use any dosage of drug between 1 and 3 mg/kg. For an individual animal (e.g. a 100 kg calf) this dosage range of 1–3 mg/kg would result in a range of potential doses (the *dose range*) of between 100 and 300 mg of drug. The dose range (e.g. 100 –300 mg for a 100 kg calf) is determined by calculating the lowest possible dose and the highest possible dose using the low and high value of the dosage range (1–3 mg/kg).

By having a dosage range and a range of potential doses, the veterinary professional can adjust the dose to accommodate the specific need of the animal (e.g. a very sick animal may get the higher dose within the dosage range and a less sick animal a lower dose). Or the veterinarian may select a dose that translates conveniently into whole tablets or capsules, eliminating the need to break tablets or use only a portion of a capsule. For example, in the case of a dosage range of 1–3 mg/kg for a 10 kg animal, the dose range would be 10–30 mg of drug. If the drug comes in 25 mg tablets, then a single whole tablet of 25 mg can be used as the administered dose because it fits within the calculated dose range of 10–30 mg.

Note that the doses are *not* usually listed as a volume (e.g. 5 mL, 15 cc) or as a number of dosage forms (e.g. 6 tablets, 2 capsules). The reason for this is because a drug may be produced by multiple manufacturers each using a different concentration of drug in their vials (e.g. Company A produces a product with 10 mg of drug per mL of liquid and Company B produces a product with 40 mg of drug per mL of liquid) or a different strength or concentration of other dosage forms (e.g. 50 mg tablet versus a 100 mg tablet, 250 mg capsule versus a 500 mg capsule). Thus, if the dose is listed only as "5 cc" or "one tablet", the veterinary professional cannot legitimately know how much mass (mg) of the drug is to be administered to the patient. The only time a dose may be listed as "one tablet," "two capsules," or "5 mL" is if the strength or concentration of the dosage form is also listed. For example, it would be a correct to say, *"two of the 100 mg ampicillin capsules* every 8 hours for 10 days."

7.1.2   The Dosage Regimen: The Route of Administration

The route of administration is the pathway by which a drug is administered to the body. For example, a drug may be administered via a needle into the vein (IV) or by having the patient swallow the medication by mouth (PO or per os). The common abbreviations used in veterinary medicine to describe routes of administration are listed in Table 7.1.

It is acceptable to write the route of administration as capital letters with periods (e.g. "I.M.") or without periods (e.g. "IM"). As a general rule, the use of uppercase or capitalized letters results in fewer

Table 7.1 Common abbreviations used in veterinary medicine to describe routes of administration

Route of administration	Description	Abbreviation
by mouth/per os	placed into the mouth and swallowed	PO
intravenous	given into the vein	IV
intramuscular	given into skeletal muscle	IM
intradermal	given into the epidermal layers of the skin	ID
intraperitoneal	given into the abdominal cavity	IP[a]
subcutaneous	given underneath the skin	SC or SQ[b]
per rectum	placed into rectum (like a suppository)	PR
right eye (*oculus dexter*)	placed into the right eye	OD[c]
left eye (*oculus sinister*)	placed into the left eye	OS
both eyes (*oculus uterque*)	placed into both eyes	OU
right ear (*auris dextra*)	placed into the right eye	AD[c]
left ear (*auris sinistra*)	placed into the left eye	AS
both ears (*auris utraque*)	placed into both eyes	AU

a   In human medicine IP could be confused with a number of other routes of administration (intrapleural, intraprostatatic), so the standard abbreviation for intraperitoneal listed in the standards of the US Food and Drug Administration is "I-PERITON." However, because these other IP routes are rarely used in veterinary medicine, IP typically means to administer the drug "into the peritoneal cavity." If there is any risk for confusion, however, the whole word should be written out on the drug order.

b   The use of the abbreviation "SQ" is a type of slang and not recognized by the US Food and Drug Administration as a standardized abbreviation for subcutaneous administration of drug. However, "SQ" is widely used in veterinary clinical practice and the veterinary technician should be aware of its use.

c   The use of OD and AD for right eye and ear respectively is generally discouraged because the lowercase versions ("od" and "ad") can be easily misinterpreted if handwritten, potentially resulting in aural (ear) medication being accidentally placed in the eye. The same can be said for the use of OS, AS and OU, AU abbreviations.

communication mistakes than lowercase letters, especially if the letters are handwritten. For example, the letter "o" can easily be mistaken for the letter "a" when handwritten and in the case of medications used in the eyes or ears, this can result in ear medications (e.g. "ad," "as," "au" routes) being administered into the eye ("od," "os," "ou") with potentially injurious effects on the cornea of the eye. Even uppercase abbreviations can be confused if poorly handwritten: a poorly written intradermal ("ID") route could be mistaken for the intraperitoneal ("IP") route. Regardless of whether a route is written in uppercase or lowercase, if there is any question about what has been written, follow the "4-A rule": "Always, always, always ask!"

In addition to the terms and abbreviations listed in Table 7.1, there are other terms used to describe the dosage regimen's route of administration. *Parenterally administered* drugs are those drugs administered by any injection (e.g. IM, IV, SQ, etc.). The term "parenteral" is derived from "para," which means "along side of," "beside," or "apart from," and "enteral," which refers to the intestinal tract. Thus, "parenterally administered" drugs are given "outside" of the intestinal tract in the area between the intestinal tract and the surface of the skin. In contrast, *enteral administered* drugs are given by mouth (PO), sublingually (under the tongue), or per rectum (into the rectrum). *Topically administered* or *topically applied* drugs are those that are applied to the surface of the skin. Intravenous drugs may be administered as an *IV bolus* or *IV push*, meaning that all of the liquid dose is administered at once, as opposed to an *IV infusion* or *constant rate infusion* (CRI), which is administration of the drug over a prolonged period of time.

7.1.3 The Dosage Regimen: The Dose Interval

The third component of the dosage regimen is the *dose interval*. The dose interval is the amount of time between each dose administration. It can be expressed as the time between each dose (e.g. every 12 hours [q12h]) or as a dose frequency (e.g. three times a day [t.i.d.]). Letters can be uppercase or lowercase and it is allowable to use periods or not use periods with the letters of the abbreviations. Table 7.2 shows the common abbreviations used in veterinary medicine to describe the dosing interval.

Table 7.2 Common abbreviations used in veterinary medicine to describe the dosing interval

Abbreviation	Description/Latin derivation	Example
q or Q	every/*quaque*	q.8.h. = every 8 hours
h or H	hour	q.6.h. = every 6 hours
d or D	day/*die*	q2d = every 2 days
s.i.d.*a*	once daily/*semel in die*	50 mg s.i.d. = 50 mg daily
b.i.d.	twice daily/*bis in die*	60 gr b.i.d. = 60 gr twice daily
t.i.d.	three times daily/*ter in die*	5 mg t.i.d. = 5 mg three times daily
q.i.d.	four times daily/*quater in die*	2 mg q.i.d. = 2 mg four times daily
q.o.d.*b*	every other day	1 tab q.o.d. = 1 tablet every other day
prn or PRN	as needed/*pro re nata*	Give one 200 mg tablet PRN
STAT	immediately/*statim*	Give 0.1 mg epinephrine IV STAT

a Neither "s.i.d." nor "SID" are recognized as a legitimate abbreviations in human medicine or pharmacy. Most pharmacists who work with veterinarians understand the terms, but it can cause confusion if a client is filling a prescription that uses the "s.i.d." abbreviation. Although "q.d." (every day) can be used in place of "s.i.d.," "q.d." can be confused with "q.i.d." (four times daily) and therefore writing out the words "every day" is preferred to using "q.d." so as to avoid confusion.

b "q.o.d." is a "slang" abbreviation that can still be found being used in veterinary medicine. However, as a general rule it should be avoided because it is not a standard interval abbreviation, it is not universally recognized, and it may be confused with "q.i.d." (four times daily). The official abbreviation for "every other day" is "q.a.d." and derives from the Latin *quoque alternis die*.

7.2 The Dosage Form

In addition to the dosage regimen (dose, route, interval, duration), drug orders may also specify the dosage form to be used to administer the medication. The dosage form of the medication is the physical form that contains the medication to be administered to the patient. Dosage forms include solids, liquids, semi-solid gels or ointments, or inhaled gas (e.g. bronchodilator inhalers or anesthetic agents). The common abbreviations used to describe dosage forms in veterinary medicine are shown in Table 7.3.

The words "*sustained release*," "*extended release*," or "*controlled release*" may be used to describe the dosage form. These terms indicate that the dosage form, usually a tablet or capsule, releases the drug slowly over an extended period of time as the dosage form passes along the intestinal tract, thus providing a slower more protracted release of the drug rather than the more immediate release of a drug found in a standard tablet or capsule dosage formulation. Several medications used in veterinary medicine are manufactured in both sustained release and regular release formulations, thus, it is important to clearly discriminate which release formulation of drug is being ordered as these different dosage forms will have different dose intervals.

Table 7.3 Common abbreviations used to describe dosage forms

Abbreviation	Description/Latin derivation	Example
tab	Tablet/*tabella*	3 tab t.i.d. = 3 tablets three times daily
cap or caps	Capsule/*capsula*	1 cap q6h = 1 capsule every 6 hours
sol[a]	Solution/*solutio*	5 mg/mL sol = 5 milligrams per milliliter solution
susp	Suspension	1 mL 3% susp = 1 milliliter of the 3% suspension
syr	syrup/*syrupus*	1 tsp cough syr = 1 teaspoon cough syrup
elix[b]	elixir	2 mL 15 gr elix = 2 milliliters of the 15 grain elixir
oint[c]	ointment	apply oint PRN = apply ointment as needed
gtt	drops/*guttae*	2 gtt OU q12h = 2 drops in both eyes every 12 hours
amp	ampule	1 amp IV STAT = 1 ampule intravenously immediately

a   the abbreviation "liq" may also be used as an abbreviation for a solution and is derived from the Latin *liquor*.
b   "elixir" and "tincture" ("tr," "tinc," "tinct") are alcohol solutions of drugs. These terms are rarely used in veterinary medicine today to describe dosage forms but were widely used in the past. Some dosage forms may still be labeled as an "elixir" or "tincture," but they are typically described in drug orders just as "solutions."
c   "oint" is a non-standard abbreviation, but is still used in veterinary medicine. The official abbreviation for ointment is "ung" and derived from the Latin *unguentum* for ointment.

7.3   The Best Practices for Writing Drug Orders

There are certain rules in writing drug orders that should be followed to reduce the risk for error. Previously, we introduced the rule about always including a zero in the ones place for any decimal number less than one (e.g. use "0.5" instead of ".5"). Here are other rules for writing drug orders or prescriptions that should be followed to reduce confusion, ambiguity, or errors:

- Do not use decimal points if they are not needed. Instead of writing "2.0", just write "2" and leave out the ".0". This reduces the risk of the "2.0" being read as "20".
- Avoid using decimal points by converting the number to its equivalent in a different unit. For example, instead of using "0.1 g" use "100 mg".
- As mentioned in the previous chapter on decimal multiplication and division, do not use trailing zeros on decimal numbers. Use "0.8" instead of "0.800".
- Abbreviations for units (e.g. kg, mL, cc) are never pluralized (do not add an "s" to the end). But when the unit names are written out, they are pluralized for any value greater than 1 (e.g. "30 kilograms").
- Units when written out fully are written in lowercase; the first letter is not capitalized unless at the beginning of a sentence. The exceptions are the temperature units Celsius and Fahrenheit.
- Whenever possible, write directions in full English and stick to using the more common Latin abbreviations stated in this text. There are hundreds of other Latin abbreviations used by physicians and pharmacists besides those listed in this textbook, but they may not be understood by veterinary professionals because they are not commonly used in veterinary medicine.
- "When in doubt, write it out!"
- Use permanent ink if handwriting drug orders on paper. Drug orders constitute part of the medical record and, as such, the medical record and the drug orders contained within it are a legal document. Corrections on a paper medical record or drug order should be indicated by a single line through the corrected part, the correction clearly written, and the initials of the individual making the correction written next to the correction. Never erase or completely block out a correction on a paper medical record or drug order as that is a violation of the integrity of the medical record and would be called into question should the record ever be used for legal purposes. Electronic medical records typically keep a log of any changes made to the medical record in order to maintain the integrity of the record as a legal document.

7.3.1 Handling Unclear Drug Orders

With the advent of electronic medical record systems, much of the confusion and errors that arose from misinterpretation of handwritten instructions or drug orders has gone away. Still, not all communication is performed electronically and it is not uncommon for a drug order to be hastily scrawled on a scrap piece of paper prior to it being formally recorded in the patient's electronic medical record. Unfortunately, handwritten drug orders can sometimes be barely legible or some abbreviation is used in the electronic medical record with which the veterinary technician is not familiar.

In these situations: do not guess what is written or stated in the drug order; *always confirm!* It is much easier to handle a simple question *before* the medication is given than to counteract an adverse drug reaction or overdose *after* the drug is administered. As a veterinary professional the care of the patient comes before any self-concern over how we think we may look if we have to ask for clarification because we are unable to read the handwriting or decipher the meaning of the electronic drug order. When in doubt, always confirm.

7.4 Understanding the Drug Label: The Drug Names

The medication label affixed to any regulated drug contains critical information required by the Food and Drug Administration (FDA) and needed for accurately carrying out drug orders. Additionally, the label also contains important information about the nature of the drug, warnings for handling the drug (if needed), and how the drug should be stored. The veterinary technician needs to know how to read the drug label to assure that the proper medication is selected for the patient and that it is administered in an appropriate and safe manner.

On most drug containers (bottles, boxes, packages), the drug is usually identified by two different names. In the example shown in Figure 7.1, there is a capitalized name ("Rimadyl") in large print and another smaller name ("carprofen").

The larger, and typically more prominent, name on the label is the *proprietary name*, *brand name*, or *trade name*. "Proprietary" means relating to an owner or ownership. Thus, the proprietary name is the name owned by one drug company. This name usually has either a circled "R" (®) after it, indicating the drug's name is registered as belonging solely to this particular drug company, or it has a trademark symbol (TM), indicating that the drug name is not yet registered but the company is staking claim to the particular drug name until it is officially registered. *Brand name* is the same as proprietary name. Although the *trade name* is usually thought of as the same as the proprietary name, the trade name can also legally apply to names, slogans, symbols, pictures, or other images that identify the drug as belonging to a particular drug company. For the purposes of this text, proprietary name, brand name, and trade name will be considered to be synonymous.

The proprietary name is a proper noun (like "Steve," "Pam," "Boston,", etc.), and therefore it is capitalized. In most cases, the proprietary name on the label is the larger and more noticeable

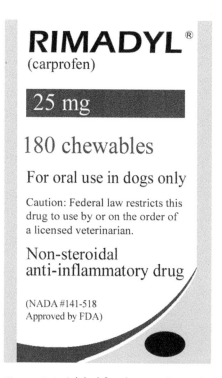

RIMADYL®
(carprofen)

25 mg

180 chewables

For oral use in dogs only

Caution: Federal law restricts this drug to use by or on the order of a licensed veterinarian.

Non-steroidal anti-inflammatory drug

(NADA #141-518
Approved by FDA)

Figure 7.1 A label for the veterinary drug Rimadyl

of the two names because this is the name the marketing department selected for the drug and thus is part of the "drug name recognition" strategy used to sell the drug product. Another company manufacturing the exact same drug would have to create a different proprietary or trade name for its product. Therefore, for common veterinary drugs like penicillin, there may be two, three, or a dozen proprietary names for that drug. Table 7.4 shows examples of different trade names of one commonly used drug.

Table 7.4 Example of proprietary names for the veterinary sedative-analgesic drug xylazine

Drug name	Proprietary name	Manufacturer
xylazine	Rompun® (original product)[a]	Bayer
xylazine	Xylaject®	Dopharma
xylazine	AnaSed®	Akorn Animal Health
xylazine	TranquiVed	VEDCO
xylazine	XylaMed™	Bimeda
xylazine	Thiazine 100	Nature Vet Products

a   The original or parent drug formulation is the first formulation of the drug to be patented, manufactured, and marketed. The company that patents the original drug formulation has a period of time specified by law during which they are the only company that can manufacture the drug. After that patent period expires, any other company can manufacture or produce the same drug. These secondary drugs are called *generic equivalents* and are often less expensive than the original parent drug product because the companies that manufacture generic equivalents did not have to invest millions of dollars into the original development, testing, and approval of their product in the way that the original drug company did.

The second, smaller, name on the label, usually written in lowercase letters, is called the *nonproprietary* or *generic* name because it is the name of the active ingredient of the drug. This active ingredient name is not owned by one particular company and therefore is "nonproprietary" ("not owned by"). Unlike the proprietary name, the nonproprietary name is usually not capitalized because it is not a proper noun. In Table 7.4 the nonproprietary name for each of those brand drugs is xylazine. In Figure 7.1, "carprofen" is the nonproprietary or generic name for Rimadyl®. Because different pharmacies and veterinary hospitals often purchase drugs from different sources, it is not unusual for different proprietary or brand names of drugs to be found in different veterinary facilities. Hence, it is good standard medical practice to always use the *nonproprietary drug* name in drug orders to avoid confusion about which drug is to be used (i.e. use the name "xylazine" in the drug order, not "Rompun®").

Occasionally, only a nonproprietary name will be listed on the drug label and there will be no brand name. The nonproprietary or generic name must *always* be listed on the label because it is the name of the active ingredient in the drug. However, when a drug has been around for many years and has been manufactured by many different companies, each with its own proprietary name, the market may be crowded with multiple proprietary or brand names and there is no marketing advantage to create yet another new brand name should another drug company choose to manufacture yet another generic form of the drug. Thus, many drug companies that manufacture "old" drugs simply list the active ingredient (e.g. "xylazine" or "carprofen") as the nonproprietary name on the label. The same can be seen for common human medications such as "aspirin" or "acetaminophen" which are often packaged as generic named products for large chain stores like Walgreens, CVS Pharmacies, etc.

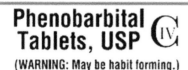

Phenobarbital Tablets, USP ℂⱽ

(WARNING: May be habit forming.)

30 mg

Ŗ Only

1000 TABLETS

Figure 7.2 Example of USP marking on a drug label

Some product labels that only have the generic, nonproprietary name will also have the initials "USP" written after the nonproprietary name (e.g. "phenobaribital USP") as shown in Figure 7.2. The USP refers to the *United States Pharmacopeia*. The USP is a nonprofit organization established in 1820 as the first attempt to identify safe medications. Today, USP sets standards for what constitutes an acceptable quality of medications that would be allowed to be sold in the United States. These USP quality standards include regulations that govern the manufacture of drugs that eventually are intended to be sold in the USA even if the raw drug material or the drug product itself are manufactured outside of the USA. The USP designation on the label indicates that the manufacture and quality control process of the drug achieved a quality level by which the drug may be legally traded and sold in the USA. Other initials occasionally seen in place of USP are "NF," which stands for the *National Formulary*. The NF is another recognized standard similar to the USP and is used on drug labels in basically the same manner.

Although the statement was made that generic or nonproprietary drug names should be used in all drug order communication or medical records, it has to be acknowledged that certain trade or proprietary names are so well entrenched in the vocabulary of veterinary medicine that these proprietary names are used to describe any drugs with the same active ingredient. For example, the proprietary brand name Valium® (for diazepam) is so widely known and was used for so many years in veterinary medicine that "Valium" is often inaccurately used to describe any diazepam product. Therefore, it is important that the veterinary professional recognize these widely used trade names and know what nonproprietary active ingredients the misused trade name represents. Table 7.5 shows some examples of commonly used proprietary names in veterinary medicine.

Like the drugs listed in Table 7.5, most antiparasitic drugs and deworming medications are known and communicated by their trade names. It is also common for newly released drugs to be discussed among veterinary professionals in casual conversation by the drug's highly publicized trade or proprietary name. However, it is still preferred to refer to a drug in written and oral communication by its nonproprietary name for greater accuracy when writing drug orders, recording drug administration in the patient record, or in communicating with professional colleagues.

The same drug manufacturer may market multiple types of drugs, all with the company's trademark logo, patterns, font styles, and colors on the label that look remarkably similar among all of the company's products. Thus, it is possible in haste to pick up the wrong bottle and to administer the wrong drug. This risk can be significantly reduced by the "three look" method of administering drugs. This safety habit is very simple:

- look at the drug label when picking up the drug
- look at the label as you are withdrawing the drug from the bottle, and finally
- look at the label one more time as you put it back down.

By doing this "three look" procedure consciously at first, and then instinctively as the habit is established, the odds of picking up the wrong drug bottle are greatly reduced.

Table 7.5 Examples of proprietary names used to represent other drugs with the same ingredients

Proprietary name commonly used	Nonproprietary name of products it represents
Valium®	diazepam (benzodiazepine tranquilizer)
Rompun®	xylazine (sedative analgesic)
Lasix®	furosemide (diuretic)
Baytril®	enrofloxacin (antibiotic)
Clavamox®	clavulanic acid + amoxicillin (antibiotic)
Rimadyl®	carprofen (nonsteroidal anti-inflammatory drug)
Flagyl®	metronidazole (antiprotozoal, antibiotic)
Benadryl®	diphenhydramine (antihistamine)
Prozac®	fluoxetine (drug for depression, OCD behavior)
Tagamet®	cimetidine (antacid)

7.5 Understanding the Drug Label: Concentrations and Dosage Forms

As was pointed out previously, injectable drugs and tablets can come in different concentrations for liquid or injectable dosage forms, and different strengths for tablets, capsules, and other solid dosage forms. Therefore, each container of medication must have a dose strength or a concentration listed.

The concentration is most commonly listed as a mass of drug (milligrams, grams, grains, etc.) per volume (milliliter, liter, cubic centimeter, etc.) of liquid into which the drug has been dissolved or suspended. On the packaging for the injectable drug shown in Figure 7.3, the concentration of drug per volume of liquid is listed as 10 mg/mL. This tells us that for each milliliter of liquid injected into the animal, 10 mg of drug is being delivered. In addition to the concentration, the total volume of liquid contained by the bottle is usually also listed (e.g. "50 mL vial").

Figure 7.3 Drug label for a liquid dosage form

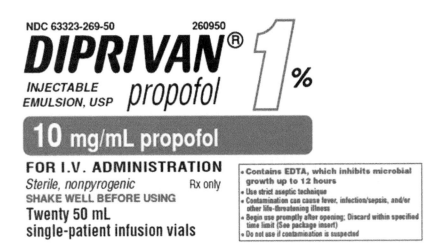

Occasionally, the drug concentration is not listed as a mass per volume unit but instead listed as a percentage. For example, the label shown in Figure 7.3 has a large "1%" listed next to the drug name, indicating that this drug concentration is a 1 *percent* solution. For this particular label the drug concentration is represented by both the percent solution (1%) and the more common mg/mL (10 mg/mL). Because a percent solution represents a mass of drug dissolved or suspended in a liquid medium, this type of concentration is also referred to as a "weight by volume" percent and may be written at "1% w/v." A concentration described by a volume of liquid mixed with another volume of liquid would be expressed as "volume by volume" or "v/v" and a "weight by weight" or "w/w" would describe a mass of powder (e.g. mg of powder) mixed with another mass of a second powder.

When only the percent solution is listed, the percent solution must be converted to the milligram per milliliter concentration in order to perform dosage calculations. The "1%" concentration in Figure 7.3 means that there is 1 g (*not* 1 mg) of drug dissolved in each 100 mL of liquid in the vial. We know this because the definition for percent solution is shown below:

$$X\% = \frac{X \text{ grams}}{100 \text{ mL}}$$

The "X" is the number used in the percent (in this example "1") and that translates directly into X g/100 mL. To convert the percent solution to the more familiar milligrams per milliliter (mg/mL), the top number X is divided by the 100, and then the number of grams is converted into milligrams using the techniques previously described in Chapter 6 for converting between metric units.

$$1\% = \frac{1\,\text{gram}}{100\,\text{mL}}$$

$$1\% = \frac{0.01\,\text{gram}}{1\,\text{mL}}$$

$$1\% = \frac{0.01\,\text{gram}}{\text{mL}} \times \frac{1000\,\text{mg}}{1\,\text{gram}}$$

$$1\% = \frac{0.01\,\cancel{\text{gram}}}{\text{mL}} \times \frac{1000\,\text{mg}}{1\,\cancel{\text{gram}}}$$

$$1\% = \frac{0.01 \times 1000\,\text{mg}}{\text{mL}}$$

$$1\% = \frac{10\,\text{mg}}{\text{mL}}$$

Table 7.6 Percent solutions with g/100 mL and mg/mL equivalents

Percent solution	Gram per 100 mL solution	mg per mL solution
1%	1 g/100 mL	10 mg/mL
5%	5 g/100 mL	50 mg/mL
25%	25 g/100 mL	250 mg/mL
0.1%	0.1 g/100 mL	1 mg/mL
0.5%	0.5 g/100 mL	5 mg/mL
4.525%	4.525 g/100 mL	45.25 mg/mL
0.0375%	0.0375 g/100 mL	0.375 mg/mL

As illustrated in Table 7.6, a shortcut for converting an "*X%*" solution to milligrams per milliliter is to remove the "%" and add a zero to the percent number. Therefore, a 5% solution is equivalent to 50 mg/mL. No matter how the veterinary professional converts a percent solution to a mg/mL concentration, the basic definition of "grams per 100 mL solution" must be memorized so it can be applied to other percent solution calculations.

Solid dosage formulations, such as tablets, caplets, and capsules, also contain a "concentration" of drug within a single dosage form and this concentration is usually referred to as the tablet's or capsule's "strength." Therefore, the concentration or "strength" for solid dosage forms might be "50 mg/tablet," "1 g/caplet," or "200 mg/capsule." It is common for a drug from one drug manufacturer to be created in a variety of different strengths or concentrations. For example, Baytril® (enrofloxacin) antibiotic tablets come in 22.7, 68, and 136 mg tablet strengths. Thus, a drug order of "1 tab Baytril q8h" would be impossible to fill accurately unless the concentration (strength) of the "1 tab" was defined in the drug order (e.g. "1 tab 22.7 mg Baytril q8h").

Notice the drug label for Baytril shown in Figure 7.4 lists the drug dosage formulation as "tablets." Each drug package will state the dosage formulation as a type of liquid dosage form (solution, suspension, tincture, elixir, "injectable") or a solid dosage form (tablets, capsules). Sometimes the dosage form itself is considered to be unique enough that the manufacturer may apply for a patent or register a name for the dosage form like "Flavor-tabs®" found in some antiparasitic drug tablets.

The dosage formulation listed on the label also conveys information about how the drug is to be used. For example, if the drug is listed as an "elixir," it is an alcohol-based liquid dosage form meant to be taken internally (e.g. phenobarbital elixir for seizure control), but if it is listed as a "tincture," it is an alcohol-based liquid dosage form most likely meant to be applied topically (e.g. iodine tincture for disinfection). A "solution" is an orally administered medication or an injectable liquid that may be given intravenously. A "suspension" is an orally administered medication or an injectable liquid that can be given IM or SQ, but is never given

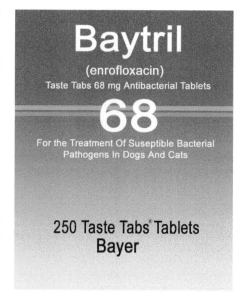

Figure 7.4 Drug label for Baytril (enrofloxacin)

intravenously because the drug is only suspended as particles floating in the liquid and if injected IV could cause vascular inflammatory reactions. An "ointment" is a semisolid dosage form that melts at body temperature and so ointments are usually applied topically (e.g. ointment for ear infections), while a "paste" is a semisolid dosage form that retains its shape at body temperature and is more commonly administered orally (e.g. equine deworming medications).

The dosage formulation may also describe other characteristics that tell something about how a drug interacts with the body or how it should be used. For example, the "sustained release" formulation mentioned previously means that the drug will be given less frequently than a drug that is in a "regular" release formulation because the sustained released medication formulation releases the drug over a longer time. A drug listed as an "enteric-coated" tablet means that the drug is protected from the harsh stomach acid and does not begin to dissolve until it passes from the stomach into the intestine.

Injectable drugs whose dosage form is described as a "vial" are usually small glass bottles with a rubber stopper that allows medication to be withdrawn more than once, using a needle. The exception to this would be the "single-dose vial" commonly used with vaccines. "Ampules," on the other hand, are small glass bottles from which contents are extracted by snapping off the smaller neck part of the ampule and using all the contents at one time.

In addition to listing the dosage form, the drug label lists the total number of units of the dosage form contained within the package. For example, for the drug in Figure 7.4, the total number of tablets contained in the bottle is 250. As described previously, liquid dosage forms usually have the total volume of liquid drug within the vial. The total number of tablets contained within a package or the total volume of liquid held within a bottle or vial is critical information for determining the amount of drug ingested and the potential toxicity if an animal or a child eats all the contents of the bottle or package.

7.6 Understanding the Drug Label: Regulatory Label Information

Notice that the drug shown in Figure 7.4 contains the statement "For the treatment of susceptible bacterial pathogens in dogs and cats." This information briefly describes the purpose for which the drug has been approved *and* the species in which the drug is approved for use. The FDA-approved purpose for the drug is called the drug's *indication*. Thus the drug in Figure 7.4 is *indicated* for treating infections caused by bacteria likely to be inhibited or killed by this drug.

The Center for Veterinary Medicine (CVM) is the branch of the FDA that is charged with regulating veterinary drug approval. When a veterinary drug manufacturer does the required testing to gain FDA approval and permission to market the drug in the USA, the manufacturer's drug label must state in which species the drug is approved for use (e.g. dog, cat, horse, beef cattle). The use of this drug in any species other than the approved species listed on the label is called *extra-label* or *off-label* use of the drug. Because veterinarians do not have FDA approved drugs available to treat all diseases in all species (especially species that are not common domesticated species), extra-label use of drugs frequently takes place. Under the requirements of Animal Medicinal Drug Use Clarification Act (AMDUCA), veterinarians may legally prescribe drugs in an extra-label manner as long as certain conditions are met. These restrictions on extra-label use are designed to reduce the risk of drug residues remaining in meat or milk which might be ingested by humans. Thus, the extra-label use of drugs in small animal practice is not very restricted since these animals are not traditionally used as human food in the USA. However, any extra-label use of drugs in food-producing animals (cattle, pigs, poultry, sheep, dairy goats) must

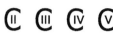

Figure 7.5 Typical warning label for restricting drug use from animals to be used for human food

conform to AMDUCA regulations to avoid residues of these untested drugs from ending up in the food people eat. If a drug is specifically designated *not* be administered to animals that could potentially be used for human food, a warning label will often be included on the drug container. An example is shown in Figure 7.5.

7.6.1 Controlled Substances and Prescription Labeling

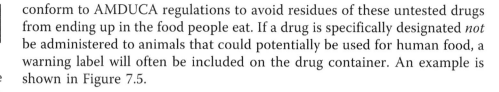

Figure 7.6 Controlled substance ratings

The label will also alert the veterinary professional to warnings if the drug requires special handling by law or for safety reasons. The presence of a large "C" plus a Roman numeral II, III, IV, or V indicates that the drug is considered a *controlled substance* (a potentially abusive substance also called a *schedule drug*) and therefore requires special record keeping and storage based upon which Roman numeral is listed. These symbols are shown in Figure 7.6. As a general rule, the lower the Roman numeral, the more abuse potential the drug has and the greater the restrictions and record keeping required. Therefore, strong opioid drugs like morphine sulfate (a C-II drug) or hydrocodone (a C-III drug) will have a much greater potential abuse than a C-IV drug like butorphanol. For further details on how controlled substances need to be stored and recorded, see a textbook on pharmacy procedures or veterinary pharmacology.

7.6.2 Prescription, Legend, and Over-The-Counter Label Indicators

The drug label also designates whether the drug can only be dispensed by order of a licensed veterinarian or a physician, or if the drug is available for purchase without a prescription as an "over-the-counter" (OTC) drug. A restriction on the availability of a drug for purchase may be stated on the label by the phrase "Caution: Federal law restricts this drug to use by or on the order of a licensed veterinarian." or by the "℞" symbol, which looks like a capital "R" with an smaller "x". The phrase restricting dispensing of the drug is called "the legend," and a drug with this phrase on its label is referred to as a "legend drug." The ℞ symbol on a legend drug bottle comes from the abbreviation for the Latin word "*recipere*," which means "take" or "take thus." Legend drugs cannot legally be made available to the public for purchase OTC. Aspirin is an OTC anti-inflammatory drug available in the aisles of grocery or drug stores, but carprofen is a legend anti-inflammatory drug and only available by prescription or veterinarian's drug order. In a veterinary hospital, the veterinarian is the only one who may prescribe legend drugs or drugs with the ℞ symbol.

Besides the controlled substances which are always legend drugs, other legend drugs would include potent antibiotics, strong pain relief medications, anesthetic agents, drugs that could potentially do harm to a patient or the person administering the drug if administered incorrectly, or drugs with significant side effects or risk for adverse reactions. OTC drugs are generally those drugs with no significant abuse potential, few significant side effects, easy to administer correctly, or otherwise very unlikely to produce harm as this reduces the liability risk of the drug manufacturer. If the manufacturer perceives there is a risk of injury from normal administration of its product, the drug usually acquires a legend or prescription restriction.

7.7 Understanding the Drug Label: Hazards, Storage, and Expiration Dates

Drugs that have a significant potential health hazard risk to either the person administering the drug or the patient are required to have a caution statement or a warning statement on the label. If the important cautionary information is too much to be contained on the drug label, the listing on the label will direct the reader to read the "package insert" or the "prescribing information" that is attached to, or packaged with, the drug. The veterinary technician should always become familiar with such information before handling and administering the drug.

| Pregnant women should not handle; handle with caution in humans with asthma and women of childbearing age. |
| Note to physician: This compound is an acetylcholinesterase inhibitor. The antidote is atropine. |
| Tablets identified 54 783 Do not use unless tablets carry this identification |

Figure 7.7 Examples of warning labels

Other warnings may include species restrictions, as described previously, cautions about route of administrations ("For oral use only," "For intravenous infusion only," "Restricted to topical use only"), abuse potential ("Warning: May be habit forming"), appearance of the drug ("Do not use if product is discolored"), or even notes to human healthcare providers that will help them treat children or adults who accidentally ingest, or come in contact with, the drug.

High abuse potential drugs that are dispensed as tablets, caplets, or capsules may have a code number listed on the label that corresponds to a code number imprinted on the dosage form itself, a picture of the dosage form, and the warning that the drug should not be used if the description on the label does not exactly match the appearance of the contents. This warning originates from the illegal practice of removing legitimate abuse drugs from a container to sell on the street and then replacing them with look-alike placebo "sugar pills" that have no effect. Examples of additional warning labels are shown in Figure 7.7.

7.7.1 Storage Information on the Label

Often the package or label has information about how the drug should be stored. This information is often printed on one of the sides of the box the bottle or vial came in or on the side of the bottle itself. For example, on boxes of Baytril (enrofloxacin), two statements sum up the key storage warnings: "Protect from direct sunlight. Do not freeze."

Storage information should be followed closely as temperature fluctuations can change the physical form of the drug, either degrading the effectiveness of the drug or changing the absorption characteristics of the drug. For example, freezing and thawing injectable penicillin G suspensions may change the crystal size of the drug, resulting in a drug that is much more painful when injected and absorbed more erratically. Drugs that are stored in the "practice truck" used by large animal and equine ambulatory veterinarians are especially susceptible to environmental exposure and variable storage conditions if the truck is parked outside on cold nights, hot days, or in garages that are not climate controlled.

7.7.2 Expiration Dates

Since 1979, all manufacturers of medications are required to stamp the expiration date on each container of a drug. This is the date that manufacturers can guarantee the full potency and safety of their drug. A large study done by the US military on drugs that had been stockpiled in anticipation for later use found that even drugs several years out of date were still perfectly good. However, the use of expired drugs can constitute a legal liability to the veterinarian should the patient experience an adverse drug reaction or not respond effectively to the treatment. Drug manufacturers will not stand behind their product used after that expiration date. A drug can lose some potency ("strength") after its expiration date, but this is a relatively slow process and the degree of drug degradation depends on the type of medication and under what conditions it is used or stored. Therefore, the safe and legal rule of thumb is that once a drug is beyond its expiration date, it should no longer be used in veterinary patients.

7.8 Chapter 7 Practice Problems

1 For each of the following written drug orders, identify the drug, the dose, the dose interval, and the route of administration:

A) "Give 50 mg of diphenhydramine by mouth three times a day."
B) "Over the next two days I want this animal to get medicated every 12 hours with ampicillin. Give 300 mg and give it subcutaneously."

2 Convert the following abbreviations into their indicated units (abbreviated):

A) q6h = _____.i.d.
B) t.i.d. = q _____ h
C) EOD = q _____ d
D) q.i.d. = q _____ h
E) q12h = _____.i.d.

3 Write out the meaning of the abbreviations used in each of the following drug orders:

A) amoxicillin tabs 50 mg, 1 tab q8h PO
B) aspirin 125 gr PO prn
C) acepromazine 15 mg, 1 tab b.i.d. prn PO
D) neomycin oint, apply AU q4h for 7 d
E) tobramycin ophthalmic drops, 2 gtt q2h OD
F) methylprednisolone, 20 mg SQ q2d for 10 d
G) ampicillin, 120 mg t.i.d. IM
H) phenobarbital elix, 30 gr po qd

4 Answer the following questions from the information contained on the drug label in Figure 7.8:

A) What is the trade name of this drug?
B) What is the generic or nonproprietary name of this drug?
C) What is the active ingredient?
D) What is the concentration of drug in each unit of the dosage form?
E) Is this a controlled substance? How do you know?
F) Is this a prescription drug or an OTC drug? How do you know?

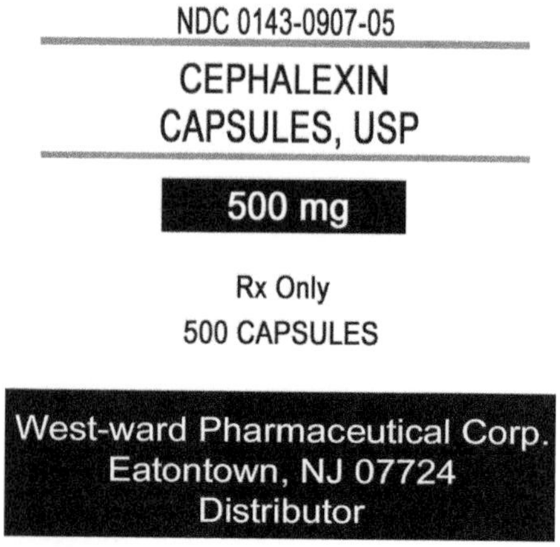

5 Answer the following questions from the information contained on the drug label in Figure 7.9:

A) Does this drug appear to have a trade name? Explain how you determined this.
B) What is the generic or nonproprietary name of this drug?
C) What does USP mean?

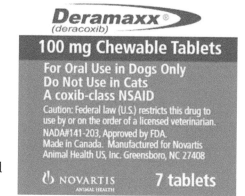

Deramaxx®
(deracoxib)
100 mg Chewable Tablets
For Oral Use in Dogs Only
Do Not Use in Cats
A coxib-class NSAID
Caution: Federal law (U.S.) restricts this drug to use by or on the order of a licensed veterinarian.
NADA#141-203, Approved by FDA.
Made in Canada. Manufactured for Novartis Animal Health US, Inc. Greensboro, NC 27408
Ů NOVARTIS
ANIMAL HEALTH
7 tablets

Figure 7.8

NDC 0143-0907-05

CEPHALEXIN
CAPSULES, USP

500 mg

Rx Only
500 CAPSULES

West-ward Pharmaceutical Corp.
Eatontown, NJ 07724
Distributor

Figure 7.9

D) Is this drug available for OTC use? How do you know?

E) Is this a controlled substance? How do you know?

6 List the following percent solutions in the corresponding units:

A) 5% = _____ g/100 mL

B) 0.3% = _____ g/100 mL

C) 7.25% = _____ mg/mL

D) 21.7% = _____ mg/mL

E) 0.02% = _____ mg/mL

Section III

Dose Calculations

8

Basic Dose Calculations

OBJECTIVES

The student will be able to:

1) convert an animal's weight from pounds to kilograms and vice versa,
2) calculate the individual dose for an animal,
3) determine the number of dose form units to administer per dose to an animal,
4) determine the total number of dose form units to be dispensed over the span of a dosage regimen, and
5) read and interpret the markings on syringes in order to properly fill a syringe with the appropriate volume of drug.

Once the basic mathematical manipulations to find the unknown X are understood and the components of the dosage regimen, including abbreviations, have been mastered, we can calculate the dose for the patient. In this chapter, we will concentrate on the basic dose calculation method and then apply it to filling a hypodermic syringe with the appropriate amount of medication.

8.1   The Basic Steps in Dose Calculation

In calculating a dose, three pieces of information are always needed:

1) the weight of the animal,
2) the dosage (amount of drug per weight of animal), and
3) the concentration of the drug in the dose form (milligrams per milliliter, milligrams per tablet, etc.).

Weight of the animal is the body weight expressed in pounds (lb), kilograms (kg), or sometimes grams (g). Accurate body weight is required, especially for drugs that have toxic principles (e.g. some antifungal agents, some cardiovascular drugs, and chemotherapeutic agents for cancer treatment). It is important to note that a hospitalized animal's weight can vary significantly over the span of its hospitalization if it does not eat as it normally should or is not getting its normal amount of exercise due to its condition. The hydration status of an animal can also significantly affect the measured body weight. Thus, it is important that the veterinary technician accurately determine the body weight on a frequent basis to make sure the amount of drug the animal is receiving remains accurate.

The drug's dosage for calculating the dose will be typically provided by the veterinarian's drug orders. However, dosages are found in special books called formularies (e.g. *Plumb's Veterinary Drug Handbook*) which list drugs with their commonly used dosages and descriptions. The drug insert information included either inside of or attached to each vial or bottle of drug will contain the manufacturer's FDA approved dosage for

Medical Mathematics and Dosage Calculations for Veterinary Technicians, Third Edition. Robert Bill.
© 2019 John Wiley & Sons, Inc. Published 2019 by John Wiley & Sons, Inc.
Companion website: www.wiley.com/go/bill/calculations

the medication. Dosages can be found on the Internet; however, it is very important to verify from where these dosages were derived as some dosages may be outside of the acceptable range for certain species. Always double check an Internet-obtained dosage with a second reliable source.

Most of the dosages found in formularies, package inserts, and other sources are listed as an amount (mass) of drug per unit of body weight:

milligrams of drug per kilogram of body weight = milligrams per kilogram = mg/kg

milligrams of drug per pound of body weight = milligrams per pound = mg/lb

grains of drug per kilogram of body weight = grains per kilogram = gr/kg

grams of drug per pound of body weight = grams per pound = g/lb

On some (relatively rare) occasions, dosages are listed in "absolute" values of drug mass instead of drug mass *per unit of body weight*. For example, the estrogen compound diethylstilbestrol (DES) is listed in some formularies as "0.1–1.0 mg PO daily for 3–5 days." Note that this is *not* 0.1–1.0 mg/kg, but an absolute amount. If this dosage was incorrectly read or interpreted as 1 mg *per kilogram of body* weight, the animal would be grossly overdosed! Therefore, clinicians will sometimes circle or underline a dose like this to emphasize that it is *not* based on a "per unit body weight" amount like most dosages.

Some medications, such as chemotherapeutic agents for treating cancer or some cardiovascular medicines, have dosages listed according to *body surface area* instead of kilograms or pounds of body weight. An example would be the dosage of digoxin (a cardiovascular medication) for dogs greater than 20 kg, which is listed as 0.22 mg/m². The "m²" is "meters squared" and represents a measure of surface area of the animal's body instead of its weight. The thought behind using this method of dosing is that the "mg/m²" provides a more accurate dose for those animals that have body weights at the upper or lower end of the weight range for the species. Digoxin is a drug whose beneficial dosage is very close to the dosage that produces adverse drug reactions (toxicity or side effects). Therefore, if dosed on a milligram per pound or milligrams per kilogram basis, very small animals may receive too little drug and very large animals may receive too much drug. Tables found in veterinary pharmacology books or veterinary drug formularies will list conversions between body weight and square meters of surface area.

Remember that some dosages are listed as a *dosage range* (e.g. 5–20 mg/kg) instead of one amount of drug per unit of body weight. This range allows the veterinary professional some latitude to adjust the patient's dose to the available dose forms (e.g. 200 mg tablet, 100 mg caplet) so that the dosage form doesn't have to be split in half or otherwise altered to match the required dose. For example, if a dosage range is listed as 2–3 mg/lb, a 10 lb animal can receive any drug dose between 20 and 30 mg. If the tablet sizes for this drug come in 10, 25, and 50 mg sizes, the dosage range allows us to select the whole 25 mg tablet, thus providing more convenience for the owners or clients.

Once the information has been gathered, the steps in actually calculating the dose are:

1) Convert the units of body weight of the animal to be congruent with the unit of body weight used in the dosage (e.g. if the dosage is listed as 5 mg/lb the animal's weight must also be listed in pounds).
2) Convert the weight of the animal into the mass of drug needed for this particular animal (e.g. the 10 kg dog needs 250 mg of drug).

3) Convert the mass of drug needed by the animal into the number of dosage forms needed per dose (e.g. number of mL per dose, number of tablets per dose, etc.)
4) Determine the total number of dosage form units needed to complete the entire length of the dosage regimen (e.g. 20 tablets for 10 days).

The next sections of this chapter will go into more detail about how each of these steps are to be calculated.

8.2 Converting the Animal's Weight into the Units Needed to Calculate the Dose

Step 1 of dose calculation requires making the units of body weight between the animal and the dosage the same.

As discussed previously, the animal's weight will be most often provided in pounds or kilograms. Likewise, dosages may be listed in metric units (e.g. milligram of drug per kilogram of body weight; mg/kg) or the avoirdupois system of pounds (e.g. milligram of drug per pound of body weight; mg/lb). Until the units of weight used for the animal are the same as the units used in the dosage, the calculation cannot be performed. Therefore, conversion of units must be made between metric and nonmetric body weights.

Chapter 6 described how to convert from nonmetric to metric body weight units using the proportion method and the cancel-out method. As an example, if given that a dog weighs 44 pounds on the veterinary hospital's scale but the dosage is listed as 5 mg/kg, the body weight unit for the patient in pounds is not congruent with the body weight unit in the dosage that is in kilograms. Thus, the animal's 44 pounds must be converted to the equivalent weight in kilograms in order for the dose for to be calculated. As a quick review of both the proportion method and the cancel-out method, the 44 lb weight will be converted to its kilogram equivalent using both methods.

The proportion method sets up an equation as shown below, where the known value unit is 44 lb; the unknown X unit is the kilogram of body weight to which the pounds must be converted, and the conversion factor is the equivalency of 2.2 lb = 1 kg. Remember that in the proportional method the fractions on either side of the equal sign must have the units arranged in the same way (i.e. kilograms on top and pounds on the bottom in this case).

$$\frac{\text{unknown } X \text{ unit}}{\text{known value unit}} = \frac{\text{conversion factor with same units as unknown } X}{\text{conversion factor with same units as known value}}$$

$$\frac{X \text{ kg}}{44 \text{ lb}} = \frac{1 \text{ kg}}{2.2 \text{ lb}}$$

$$44 \text{ lb} \times \frac{X \text{ kg}}{44 \text{ lb}} = \frac{1 \text{ kg}}{2.2 \text{ lb}} \times 44 \text{ lb}$$

$$\cancel{44 \text{ lb}} \times \frac{X \text{ kg}}{\cancel{44 \text{ lb}}} = \frac{1 \text{ kg}}{2.2 \text{ lb}} \times 44 \text{ lb}$$

$$X \text{ kg} = \frac{1 \text{ kg}}{2.2 \cancel{\text{ lb}}} \times 44 \cancel{\text{ lb}}$$

$$X \text{ kg} = \frac{1 \text{ kg}}{2.2} \times 44$$

$$X \text{ kg} = 20 \text{ kg}$$

44 pounds is equivalent to 20 kg. Check the 20 kg answer by plugging it into the original equation to see if both sides of the equation balance.

$$\frac{X \text{ kg}}{44 \text{ lb}} = \frac{1 \text{ kg}}{2.2 \text{ lb}}$$

$$\frac{20 \text{ kg}}{44 \text{ lb}} = \frac{1 \text{ kg}}{2.2 \text{ lb}}$$

$$\frac{0.454 \text{ kg}}{\text{lb}} = \frac{0.454 \text{ kg}}{\text{lb}}$$

Both sides of the equal sign are the same so the answer is correct.

The same answer is obtained using the cancel-out method. Remember that in the cancel-out method the unknown X is put on one side of the equation and all the other values are placed on the other side in such a way that units in the numerator (top part of the fraction) cancel out with the same units in the denominator (bottom part of the fraction), leaving only the unit of the unknown X (kilograms in this case) in the top part of the fraction or by itself.

$$\text{unknown } X \text{ unit} = \text{known value unit} \times \frac{\text{conversion factor with same units as unknown } X}{\text{conversion factor with same units as known value}}$$

$$X \text{ kg} = 44 \text{ lb} \times \frac{1 \text{ kg}}{2.2 \text{ lb}}$$

$$X \text{ kg} = 44 \text{ \cancel{lb}} \times \frac{1 \text{ kg}}{2.2 \text{ \cancel{lb}}}$$

$$X \text{ kg} = 44 \times \frac{1 \text{ kg}}{2.2}$$

$$X \text{ kg} = \frac{44 \text{ kg}}{2.2}$$

$$X \text{ kg} = 20 \text{ kg}$$

Either method of calculation arrives at the same answer, so it is a matter of personal choice which method to use. The key point is to practice doing the same method repeatedly to reduce the chances of making errors when performing these calculations.

8.3   Determining the Dose for the Patient

After the units for the animal's weight and the body weight listed in the dosage have been aligned, step two can be completed to determine the amount of mass of drug (the dose, usually expressed as milligrams of drug) this particular patient needs. The information provided for this calculation is the body weight of the patient and the dosage. Regardless of whether the proportion method or the cancel-out method is used, the unknown X for this step is the *amount of drug* this patient needs (the patient's dose). The known element in this problem is the patient's body weight. The "conversion factor" that enables us to get from body weight to mass of drug is the *dosage* (e.g. 5 mg/kg).

Assume a 20 kg (44 lb) animal needs a drug and the drug's dosage for this species is 5 mg/kg. This would be 5 mg of drug for every kilogram of the patient's body weight. The exact number of milligrams of drug to give this particular animal is then determined as shown below.

Proportion Method

$$\frac{\text{unknown } X \text{ unit}}{\text{known value unit}} = \frac{\text{conversion factor with same units as unknown } X}{\text{conversion factor with same units as known value}}$$

$$\frac{X \text{ mg}}{20 \text{ kg}} = \frac{5 \text{ mg}}{\text{kg}}$$

$$20 \text{ kg} \times \frac{X \text{ mg}}{20 \text{ kg}} = \frac{5 \text{ mg}}{\text{kg}} \times 20 \text{ kg}$$

$$\cancel{20 \text{ kg}} \times \frac{X \text{ mg}}{\cancel{20 \text{ kg}}} = \frac{5 \text{ mg}}{\text{kg}} \times 20 \text{ kg}$$

$$X \text{ mg} = \frac{5 \text{ mg}}{\cancel{\text{kg}}} \times 20 \, \cancel{\text{kg}}$$

$$X \text{ mg} = \frac{5 \text{ mg}}{} \times 20$$

$$X \text{ mg} = 100 \text{ mg}$$

Cancel-out Method

$$\text{unknown } X \text{ unit} = \text{known value unit} \times \frac{\text{conversion factor with same units as unknown } X}{\text{conversion factor with same units as kown value}}$$

$$X \text{ mg} = 20 \text{ kg} \times \frac{5 \text{ mg}}{\text{kg}}$$

$$X \text{ mg} = 20 \, \cancel{\text{kg}} \times \frac{5 \text{ mg}}{\cancel{\text{kg}}}$$

$$X \text{ mg} = 20 \times \frac{5 \text{ mg}}{}$$

$$X \text{ mg} = 20 \times 5 \text{ mg}$$

$$X \text{ mg} = 100 \text{ mg}$$

The 20 kg animal, given the drug at a dosage of 5 mg/kg, will need to receive 100 mg of the drug for a proper dose. Once the mass of drug has been determined for the patient, the next step is to determine how much of the physical dose form (tablets, liquid) must be given to the animal in order to deliver the prescribed 100 mg of drug.

8.4 Determining the Amount of Dose Forms Needed per Dose

As described in Chapters 6 and 7, dosage forms come as liquids, semi-solids, solids, and a wide variety of other dosage forms. Dosage calculations are typically only used to determine volume of liquid dosage forms or number of solid dosage forms needed per dose and to fulfill the needs for the duration of the dosage regimen. The concentration of the drug within the liquid dosage form or the amount of drug within a single unit of the solid dosage form (the strength of the tablet, capsule, etc.) is the key piece of information needed to convert from the patient's needed dose to the number of dosage forms. In the case of liquids, concentration is usually expressed as a drug mass per volume of liquid medium (e.g. 100 mg/mL, 5 g/100 mL) or as a percent solution (e.g. 2.27%, 15%). For solid dose forms the concentration is the amount of drug within one solid unit of the dosage form (e.g. 50 mg/tablet, 100 mg/capsule, 6 mg/tsp of powder).

As an example, it has been determined that a patient needs 100 mg of drug. The drug is to be administered by injection, therefore the concentration of the injectable solution must be known. The label of the drug lists a concentration of 200 mg/mL, which is the same as saying that 200 mg of drug is present in each milliliter of liquid withdrawn from the vial. The unknown X is now the number of milliliters of liquid of this drug needed to deliver 100 mg of medication, the known value is the previously calculated drug dose of 100 mg; and the conversion factor is the 200 mg/mL concentration of drug in liquid.

Proportion Method

$$\frac{\text{unknown } X \text{ unit}}{\text{known value unit}} = \frac{\text{conversion factor with same units as unknown } X}{\text{conversion factor with same units as known value}}$$

$$\frac{X \text{ mL}}{100 \text{ mg}} = \frac{1 \text{ mL}}{200 \text{ mg}}$$

$$100 \text{ mg} \times \frac{X \text{ mL}}{100 \text{ mg}} = \frac{1 \text{ mL}}{200 \text{ mg}} \times 100 \text{ mg}$$

$$\cancel{100 \text{ mg}} \times \frac{X \text{ mL}}{\cancel{100 \text{ mg}}} = \frac{1 \text{ mL}}{200 \text{ mg}} \times 100 \text{ mg}$$

$$X \text{ mL} = \frac{1 \text{ mL}}{200 \cancel{\text{ mg}}} \times 100 \cancel{\text{ mg}}$$

$$X \text{ mL} = \frac{1 \text{ mL}}{200} \times 100$$

$$X \text{ mL} = 0.5 \text{ mL}$$

Cancel-out Method

$$\text{unknown } X \text{ unit} = \text{known value unit} \times \frac{\text{conversion factor with same units as unknown } X}{\text{conversion factor with same units as known value}}$$

$$X \text{ mL} = 100 \text{ mg} \times \frac{1 \text{ mL}}{200 \text{ mg}}$$

$$X \text{ mL} = 100 \cancel{\text{ mg}} \times \frac{1 \text{ mL}}{200 \cancel{\text{ mg}}}$$

$$X \text{ mL} = 100 \times \frac{1 \text{ mL}}{200}$$

$$X \text{ mL} = \frac{100 \times 1 \text{ mL}}{200}$$

$$X \text{ mL} = 0.5 \text{ mL}$$

When the concentration is expressed as percent solutions (see Chapter 7), we have to perform an additional step in our calculations in order to change the percent solution concentration to its equivalent milligram per milliliter (mg/mL) concentration. To convert the percent solution, remember the definition of a percent solution: X% solution is equivalent to X number of grams in 100 mL of fluid. Another shortcut is to memorize that X% solution is equivalent to 10 times X mg/mL.

$$X\%\text{solution} = \frac{X \text{ grams}}{100 \text{ mL}} = \frac{X \times 10 \text{ mg}}{\text{mL}}$$

Using these definitions, a 20% solution would be equivalent to 20 g of drug/100 mL of liquid or 200 mg of drug/mL of liquid.

$$20\%\text{solution} = \frac{20 \text{ grams}}{100 \text{ mL}} = \frac{20 \times 10 \text{ mg}}{\text{mL}} = \frac{200 \text{ mg}}{\text{mL}}$$

Once the percent solution has been converted into a "mg/mL" concentration form, that concentration form is used to determine the amount of the dose form needed to deliver the dose for the patient, as described previously.

For tablets, the concentration conversion factor most commonly used is X mg/tablet, although any mass of drug (grain, grams, etc.) per solid dose form unit (capsule, caplet, measured powder, etc.) can be used. If a 20 kg animal needs 100 mg of drug and the tablet bottle lists the dosage formulation strength (concentration of tablet) as 50 mg of drug per tablet, we can calculate how many tablets are needed. Our unknown X is the number of tablets needed for the dose; the known value is the dose of drug for this animal (100 mg), and the conversion factor is the concentration of the tablets (50 mg/tablet).

Proportion Method

$$\frac{\text{unknown } X \text{ unit}}{\text{known value unit}} = \frac{\text{conversion factor with same units as unknown } X}{\text{conversion factor with same units as known value}}$$

$$\frac{X \text{ tablets}}{100 \text{ mg}} = \frac{1 \text{ tablet}}{50 \text{ mg}}$$

$$100 \text{ mg} \times \frac{X \text{ tablets}}{100 \text{ mg}} = \frac{1 \text{ tablet}}{50 \text{ mg}} \times 100 \text{ mg}$$

$$\cancel{100 \text{ mg}} \times \frac{X \text{ tablets}}{\cancel{100 \text{ mg}}} = \frac{1 \text{ tablet}}{50 \text{ mg}} \times 100 \text{ mg}$$

$$X \text{ tablets} = \frac{1 \text{ tablet}}{50 \; \cancel{\text{mg}}} \times 100 \; \cancel{\text{mg}}$$

$$X \text{ tablets} = \frac{1 \text{ tablet}}{50} \times 100$$

$$X \text{ tablets} = \frac{1 \text{ tablet} \times 100}{50}$$

$$X \text{ tablets} = 2 \text{ tablets}$$

Cancel-out Method

$$\text{unknown } X \text{ unit} = \text{known value unit} \times \frac{\text{conversion factor with same units as unknown } X}{\text{conversion factor with same units as known value}}$$

$$X \text{ tablets} = 100 \text{ mg} \times \frac{1 \text{ tablet}}{50 \text{ mg}}$$

$$X \text{ tablets} = 100 \, \cancel{\text{mg}} \times \frac{1 \text{ tablet}}{50 \, \cancel{\text{mg}}}$$

$$X \text{ tablets} = 100 \times \frac{1 \text{ tablet}}{50}$$

$$X \text{ tablets} = \frac{100 \times 1 \text{ tablet}}{50}$$

$$X \text{ tablets} = 2 \text{ tablets}$$

Although the common way to describe tablet concentrations is to say "50 mg per tablet," represented mathematically as "50 mg/tablet," the conversion factor used in this calculation is set up so that it is "1 tablet per 50 mg" and represented mathematically as "1 tablet/50 mg." If the conversion factor had been written the way people normally talk, the problem would have been set up incorrectly! Therefore, by carefully following the rules for arranging the values by their unit labels, the problem is set up the correct way and avoids an incorrect calculation resulting in a significant overdose or under dose for the patient.

Calculations for solid dosage forms often do not result in a convenient, even number of dosage forms. Instead, the calculation usually results in a fractional dose such as 2.187 tablets or 1.745 tablets. No client or veterinary technician is going to slice off 0.187 of a tablet to accurately administer a dose. As a result, fractional answers to the dose must be rounded.

Because veterinarians often prescribe human medications for veterinary patients and because human dosage formulations are typically manufactured to be conveniently dosed for 130–150 pound humans, the veterinary dose for human drugs often results in a fractional number of solid dosage forms for the veterinary patient. As a general rule, tablets should not be cut into anything less than half unless the tablet is large and scored. A scored tablet has partial cuts in the tablet that allow accurate splitting into quarters. More typically, tablets are not scored into quarters and a dose calculation requiring 1/4 or 1/8 of a tablet must be either recalculated for a different tablet strength, if available, or the calculated number of tablets per dose must be rounded to the nearest half or whole tablet. When rounding the calculated tablet dose to the nearest half or whole tablet, follow the chart in Table 8.1, which illustrates the appropriate rounding.

If the calculated tablet dose comes out to 0.25 or 0.75 tablet, the tablet dose can be rounded either to the nearest half or whole. If the drug has some significant risk of causing side effects, the veterinarian may

Table 8.1 Rounding dose appropriately to nearest half or whole tablet

Calculated tablet dose	Rounded tablet dose
up to 0.5 tablet	½ tablet
0.5 to 0.75 tablet	½ tablet
0.75 to 1 tablet	1 tablet
1 to 1.25 tablet	1 tablet
1.25 to 1.50 tablet	1½ tablet
1.50 to 1.75 tablet	1½ tablet
1.75 to 2 tablets	2 tablets

cautiously decide to round "down" to the nearest whole or half. For drugs that are not otherwise toxic, which way the dose form is rounded doesn't matter.

8.5 Determining the Number of Dosage Forms Needed to Complete the Dosage Regimen

If medication is being dispensed as tablets or liquid for the owner to administer over several days, the number of dosage forms must be calculated for dispensing. For example, if the drug order states that the animal is going to receive "2 tabs q8h for 6d," the drug order has to be deciphered and the total number of units to be dispensed determined. Although the total number of dosage form units can often be determined without writing out the problem, it is important to understand how this type of problem is set up so more complex dispensing problems can be accurately calculated.

The unknown X in this type of problem is going to be the total number of tablets, capsules, milliliters of liquid, or other dosage units to be dispensed. The known value for our calculation is the total number of doses to be used over the length of the dosage regimen. The conversion factor is the number of dosage form units per dose (in our example previously, it was determined to be two tablets *per dose*). The total number of doses (the known value in our equation) is determined by multiplying the number of doses per day by the number of days the doses are to be administered according to the drug order. In our example of "q8h for 6d," the abbreviation translates into "every 8 hours for 6 days," meaning that the dose is going to be given three times a day for six days.

$$\text{total number of doses} = \frac{\text{number of doses}}{1 \text{ day}} \times \text{number of days}$$

$$\text{total number of doses} = \frac{3 \text{ doses}}{1 \text{ day}} \times 6 \text{ days}$$

$$\text{total number of doses} = \frac{3 \text{ doses}}{1 \text{ \sout{day}}} \times 6 \text{ \sout{days}}$$

$$\text{total number of doses} = \frac{3 \text{ doses}}{} \times 6 = 18 \text{ doses}$$

Once the total number of doses that are to be administered has been determined (18 doses in this case), this value becomes the known value in using the proportional or cancel-out method to determine the unknown total number of tablets. The conversion factor for converting doses into tablets is the number of tablets *per dose*, which in this example was stated to be "2 tablets per dose."

Proportion Method

$$\frac{\text{unknown } X \text{ unit}}{\text{known value unit}} = \frac{\text{conversion factor with same units as unknown } X}{\text{conversion factor with same units as known value}}$$

$$\frac{X \text{ tablets}}{18 \text{ doses}} = \frac{2 \text{ tablets}}{\text{dose}}$$

$$18 \text{ doses} \times \frac{X \text{ tablets}}{18 \text{ doses}} = \frac{2 \text{ tablets}}{\text{dose}} \times 18 \text{ doses}$$

$$\cancel{18 \text{ doses}} \times \frac{X \text{ tablets}}{\cancel{18 \text{ doses}}} = \frac{2 \text{ tablets}}{\text{dose}} \times 18 \text{ doses}$$

$$X \text{ tablets} = \frac{2 \text{ tablets}}{\cancel{\text{dose}}} \times 18 \cancel{\text{ doses}}$$

$$X \text{ tablets} = \frac{2 \text{ tablets}}{} \times 18$$

$$X \text{ tablets} = 36 \text{ tablets}$$

Cancel-out Method

$$\text{unknown } X \text{ unit} = \text{known value unit} \times \frac{\text{conversion factor with same units as unknown } X}{\text{conversion factor with same units as known value}}$$

$$X \text{ tablets} = 18 \text{ doses} \times \frac{2 \text{ tablets}}{\text{dose}}$$

$$X \text{ tablets} = 18 \cancel{\text{ doses}} \times \frac{2 \text{ tablets}}{\cancel{\text{dose}}}$$

$$X \text{ tablets} = 18 \times \frac{2 \text{ tablets}}{}$$

$$X \text{ tablets} = 36 \text{ tablets}$$

To use the calculation with other dose form units (e.g. milliliters, capsules), the same general procedures are used replacing the "tablets" units with the appropriate dosage form per dose (e.g. milliliters per dose, caplets per dose).

8.5.1 The Most Common Mistake Made when Determining the Total Number of Units to Be Dispensed

A veterinary technician student was given the following dose order for a 39 lb dog: "Give 5 mg/kg b.i.d. for 7 d." The medication comes in 50 mg tablets. The student went about filling the order in the following manner. Can you detect where the student went wrong in figuring out the total number of tablets to be dispensed?

Step 1. The student first converted the dog's 39 lb weight to kilograms:

$$X \text{ kg} = 39 \text{ lb} \times \frac{1 \text{ kg}}{2.2 \text{ lb}}$$

$$X \text{ kg} = \frac{39 \text{ kg}}{2.2}$$

$$X \text{ kg} = 17.72\overline{72} \text{ kg}$$

$$X \text{ kg} = 17.7 \text{ kg}$$

Step 2. The dose in milligrams was calculated for a 17.7 kg dog using the 5 mg/kg dosage:

$$X \text{ mg} = 17.7 \, \cancel{\text{kg}} \times \frac{5 \text{ mg}}{\cancel{\text{kg}}}$$

$$X \text{ mg} = 17.7 \times \frac{5 \text{ mg}}{}$$

$$X \text{ mg} = 88.5 \text{ mg}$$

Step 3. The total number of doses was determined for "b.i.d. for 7d":

$$\text{total number of doses} = \frac{2 \text{ doses}}{1 \text{ day}} \times 7 \text{ days} = 14 \text{ total doses}$$

Step 4. Using the dose (86.5 mg), the student then figured the total amount of drug needed for 7 days:

$$X \text{ mg total for 7 days} = 14 \text{ doses} \times \frac{88.5 \text{ mg}}{\text{dose}}$$

$$X \text{ mg total for 7 days} = 14 \, \cancel{\text{doses}} \times \frac{88.5 \text{ mg}}{\cancel{\text{dose}}}$$

$$X \text{ mg total for 7 days} = 14 \times \frac{88.5 \text{ mg}}{}$$

$$X \text{ mg total for 7 days} = 1239 \text{ mg}$$

Step 5. The student then calculated the total number of 50 mg tablets needed to deliver 1239 mg of drug:

$$X \text{ mg total tablets for 7 days} = 1239 \text{ mg} \times \frac{1 \text{ tablet}}{50 \text{ mg}}$$

$$X \text{ mg total tablets for 7 days} = 1239 \, \cancel{\text{mg}} \times \frac{1 \text{ tablet}}{50 \, \cancel{\text{mg}}}$$

$$X \text{ mg total tablets for 7 days} = \frac{1239 \text{ tablets}}{50}$$

$$X \text{ mg total tablets for 7 days} = 24.78 \text{ tablets} = \text{rounded to 25 tablets}$$

But when the veterinary technician tried to determine how many tablets the client needed to give the patient *per dose*, the 25 total tablets did not divide evenly into the 14 doses:

$$25 \text{ tablets} \div 14 \text{ doses} = 1.7857143 \text{ tablets per dose}$$

The math was all correct! So how did this calculation we end up with such an "unusable" tablet dose?

The answer is that the veterinary technician should have converted the 88.5 mg *per dose* to the number of tablets *per dose* after Step 2 of the calculations. Obviously, if the calculated individual drug dose (88.5 mg) didn't fit evenly into a half or whole 50 mg tablet, then some awkward fraction of the 50 mg tablet was going to be needed to deliver 88.5 mg of drug. By calculating the total mass of drug needed for the entire dose regimen (1239 mg) and then dividing that into 50 mg tablets, the result produced tablet numbers in an unusable fraction of a tablet. Instead, in Step 2, the 88.5 mg *per dose* should have been rounded to the closest half or whole 50 mg tablet per dose *before* determining the total dosage forms needed for the whole dosage regimen. The "88.5 mg" represents 88.5 mg *per dose* but the "dose" unit is implied and left out of the actual calculation.

$$X \text{ tablets per dose} = 88.5 \text{ mg} \times \frac{1 \text{ tablet}}{50 \text{ mg}}$$

$$X \text{ tablets per dose} = 88.5 \; \cancel{\text{mg}} \times \frac{1 \text{ tablet}}{50 \; \cancel{\text{mg}}}$$

$$X \text{ tablets per dose} = \frac{88.5 \times 1 \text{ tablet}}{50}$$

$$X \text{ tablets per dose} = 1.77 \text{ tablets}$$

1.77 tablet is closer to 2.0 full tablets than it is to 1.5 tablets, so the number of tablets to be given *per dose* is rounded to 2 tablets. Now the total number of dispensed tablets for the 14 doses can be determined and the final total to be dispensed will divide evenly into the 14 doses:

$$X \text{ mg total tablets for 7 days} = 14 \text{ doses} \times \frac{2 \text{ tablets}}{\text{dose}}$$

$$X \text{ mg total tablets for 7 days} = 14 \; \cancel{\text{doses}} \times \frac{2 \text{ tablets}}{\cancel{\text{dose}}}$$

$$X \text{ mg total tablets for 7 days} = 14 \times 2 \text{ tablets} = 28 \text{ tablets}$$

Key point: to avoid making this dispensing mistake, the amount of drug *per dose* must be converted into the number of dose units per dose *before* determining the total dose units to be dispensed.

8.6 Determining the Cost for Dispensed Medication

Once the total number of units to be dispensed has been determined, the cost to the client must be calculated. The cost per unit (e.g. the cost of 1 cc of liquid or 1 tablet) is typically provided or posted within the hospital dispensing area. However, if only the total cost for the entire bottle or vial of drug is known, the individual unit cost can be easily determined.

$$\text{cost for one dose form unit} = \frac{\text{total cost for all dose form units}}{\text{number of dose form units}}$$

For example, if a bottle of tablets is listed as $32.00 and there are 100 tablets within the bottle, each individual tablet (one dose form unit) is $0.32 or 32 cents.

$$\text{cost for one dose form unit} = \frac{\text{total cost for all dose form units}}{\text{number of dose form units}} = \frac{\$32.00}{100 \text{ tablets}} = \frac{\$0.32}{\text{tablet}}$$

The same method would apply to determining the cost of the individual liquid dose form unit given the cost of the vial of injectable or orally administered liquid.

The total cost for the number of units dispensed would be determined by multiplying the individual cost per unit by the total number of units dispensed. For example, if 25 tablets in the previous example were dispensed, the total cost would be:

$$\text{total cost for dispensed units} = \text{number of units dispensed} \times \frac{\text{cost}}{1 \text{ unit}}$$

$$\text{total cost for dispensed units} = 25 \times \frac{\$0.32}{\text{tablet}} = \$8.00$$

Often there is a dispensing fee charged by the veterinary hospital for any drug dispensed from the hospital's pharmacy. The fee is added after the total cost of the dispensed medication has been determined.

$$\text{total cost} = \$8.00 \text{ for medication} + \$5.00 \text{ dispensing fee} = \$13.00$$

8.7 Using a Syringe with Liquid Dosage Formulations

Liquid dosage forms can be "loaded" into a syringe for administration orally or by injection. In order for the correct amount of drug to be delivered, the proper dose calculation must be performed and the correct amount of drug pulled into the syringe. Reading the syringe properly helps ensure that the proper volume of medication will be administered.

Plastic syringes used in veterinary medicine range in total capacity from small 1 cc (1 mL) syringes all the way up to large 60 cc syringes. The 3 cc syringe is the most commonly used syringe in small animal medicine to deliver vaccines and most injected medications. The 1 cc syringe is called a "tuberculin syringe" because the small single mL volume and proportionally small needle make it idea for injecting small amounts of tuberculin antigen to perform intradermal skin testing for tuberculosis. Another type of dosing syringe more often used in livestock production facilities is the multidose syringe or "dose gun," which is capable of delivering measured amounts of medication repeatedly with each squeeze of the spring-loaded trigger. Large metallic oral dosing syringes with blunted metal tips are also used to administer liquid oral medications to horses and livestock.

Plastic syringes for injection purposes are designed to be used once and then discarded into a safe, secure "sharps" container and disposed as biohazardous waste. The syringe consists of a plastic barrel into which the rubber-tipped plunger slides. The rubber tip to the plunger has two rings that create a water tight seal to keep loaded drug from leaking out along the plunger. Medication loaded into the syringe is pushed out of the syringe through the tip and into the hypodermic needle which is attached to the syringe either by pushing the needle hub onto the syringe tip (sometimes called a "slip tip" type of connection) or screwing the hub of the needle onto the syringe (the Luer threaded type of fitting, often referred to by the proprietary name Luer-Lok® syringes). The barrel of the syringe has incremental markings to indicate the volume of liquid pulled or "loaded" into the syringe.

8.7.1 Syringes in Veterinary Medicine

One special type of plastic syringe is the insulin syringe. Insulin is used to treat diabetes mellitus and is a synthesized hormone. The doses of insulin are not measured in volumes like most drugs (e.g. 5 mL or 3 cc) but are measured as "units." The unit reflects a unit of biological activity of the insulin hormone as opposed to the concentration of insulin in the liquid medium (although there is a correlation between the amount of pure insulin in each liquid volume amount and the biological activity that amount will produce). Multidose vials of insulin used in veterinary medicine typically come in standardized concentrations of 40 units/mL; however, 100 units/mL vials are standard for insulin used in human patients. Therefore, the abbreviation U-40 on either a syringe or a vial of insulin refers to the standard concentration of 40 units (U) of insulin in each mL (cc) of liquid medium. A U-100 vial of insulin (100 units in each mL of liquid medium) requires the use of a U-100 syringe for accurate administration, and U-40 insulin requires a U-40 insulin syringe. Because each insulin syringe has a volume capacity of 1 mL, the markings on the U-40 syringe range from 0 to 40, and the markings on the U-100 syringe range from 0 to 100.

Figure 8.1 illustrates the markings on the barrel of a standard 3 cc (3 mL) syringe. The markings show increments of 0.1 (one-tenth) cubic centimeter or 0.1 mL. Figure 8.2 shows a 6 cc (6 mL) syringe. Unlike the increments on the 3 cc syringe, each mark on the 6 cc syringe indicates 0.2 mL. Most larger syringes, like the 35 cc syringe shown in Figure 8.3, have 1 cc (1 mL) increments marked on the syringe barrel. While a dose of 2.3 mL would be quite easy to accurately load into a 3 cc syringe, the same 2.3 mL might be off by 0.5 mL or more if drawn into the larger 35 cc syringe. Therefore, it is important to choose a syringe with appropriate incremental barrel markings that will provide the greatest degree of accuracy for loading the liquid dose into the syringe.

Sometimes a second scale of increments besides the cc or mL may be found on the barrel of the syringe to facilitate drug dosing. For example, the image of the large 35 cc syringe in

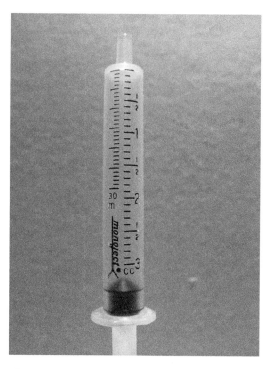

Figure 8.1 Markings on the barrel of a 3 cc (3 mL) syringe.

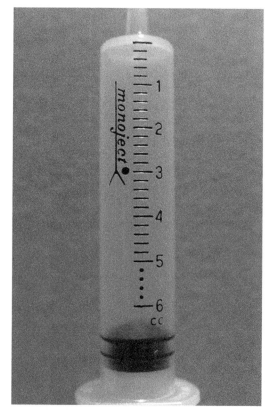

Figure 8.2 Markings on the barrel of a 6 cc (6 mL) syringe. Note the 0.2 mL increments.

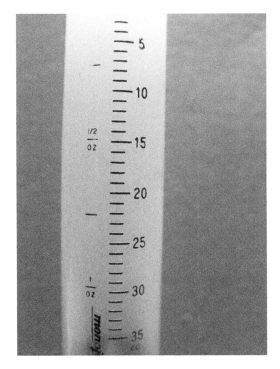

Figure 8.3 Markings on the barrel of a 35 cc (35 mL) syringe.

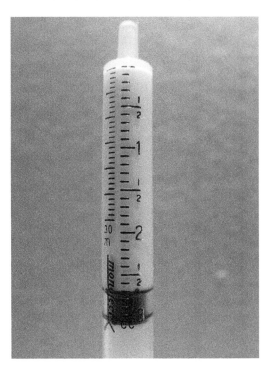

Figure 8.4 3 cc syringe filled with 2.7 cc or 2.7 mL of drug.

Figure 8.3 shows an alternate scale with markings for 1/4, 1/2, 3/4 and 1 fluid ounce. Only the 1/2 and 1 fluid ounce marks are labeled on the barrel and the fluid ounce unit is abbreviated as "oz" when it technically should be "fl oz" to differentiate it from the weight unit ounce.

8.7.2 Measuring Fluid within the Syringe

The 3 cc syringe shown in Figure 8.4 has been filled with 2.7 mL or 2.7 cc of drug. Notice how the black plunger appears to have two rings that define the top and bottom of the rubber plunger. The top ring of the plunger closest to the syringe tip defines the volume of the liquid loaded into the syringe. When drawing the drug from the vial into the syringe barrel, the volume of drug loaded is always read by the edge of the top ring of the black plunger. Sometimes, beginning students incorrectly use the bottom ring of the plunger (farther away from the hub) as the volume "indicator," resulting in less drug being delivered to the patient than was calculated to be given.

If air bubbles become mixed with the drug in the syringe barrel, the amount of drug in the syringe cannot be accurately measured since part of the syringe volume is occupied by air. In those situations, the air can be removed by holding the syringe vertically (needle end up) and firmly tapping the syringe barrel with a flick of the finger to cause the air bubbles to form one larger bubble that will rise into the hub and can be expelled with minimal drug loss.

To accurately deliver the prescribed dose of the drug, the rubber plunger of the syringe must be pushed to the hub as far as it can go. Even so, some of the drug will remain in the hub itself. This is of no consequence in determining the volume of drug to be delivered because the small volume in the hub is factored into the volume markings on the barrel. However, the veterinary professional must remember that for potentially dangerous drugs like antineoplastic, cancer-fighting drugs, the hub will hold some of this drug and there is potential for accidental exposure to the drug if the syringe is dismantled for disposal or if the syringe is flushed with air.

8.8   Chapter 8 Practice Problems

1   Convert the animal's weight to the equivalent weight in the given units:

A)   30 kg = _____ lb
B)   88 lb = _____ kg
C)   23.3 kg = _____ lb
D)   1348 lb = _____ kg
E)   238 kg = _____ lb
F)   22 lb = _____ kg
G)   100 kg = _____ lb
H)   791.6 lb = _____ kg
I)   0.4 kg = _____ lb
J)   0.85 lb = _____ kg
K)   0.0321 kg = _____ lb
L)   0.032 lb = _____ kg
M)   3092 g = _____ kg
N)   5292 g = _____ lb

2   Determine how much drug (in milligrams) each animal needs:

A)   43 lb dog; dose is 2 mg/lb = _____ mg
B)   4 kg cat; dose is 2.5 mg/kg = _____ mg
C)   21 kg dog; dose is 15 mg/lb = _____ mg
D)   11 lb cat; dose is 5 mg/kg = _____ mg
E)   896 lb horse; dose is 2 mg/kg = _____ mg
F)   0.5 kg rat; dose is 0.25 mg/kg = _____ mg
G)   8.5 lb cat; dose is 50 mg/kg = _____ mg
H)   65 lb dog; dose is 3 mg/lb = _____ mg
I)   423 lb calf; dose is 0.5 mg/kg = _____ mg
J)   150 kg sow; dose is 0.25 mg/lb = _____ mg
K)   0.75 kg guinea pig; dose is 0.35 mg/kg = _____ mg
L)   800 g bird; dose is 1.3 mg/kg = _____ mg
M)   dog with 1.2 m^2; dose is 0.75 mg/m^2 = _____ mg
N)   cat with 0.03 m^2; dose is 60 mg/m^2 = _____ mg

3   Given the patient parameter and a dosage *range*, determine the minimum dose and the maximum dose an animal could be given. For example, given that a dog weighs 10 kg and the dosage range is 2–4 mg/kg, the minimum dose that could be given to this patient would be 20 kg and the maximum dose would be 40 kg.

A)   11 kg dog; dosage range 4–10 mg/lb
       minimum dose = _____ mg, maximum dose = _____ mg
B)   0.5 kg kitten; dosage range 200–250 mg/lb
       minimum dose = _____ mg, maximum dose = _____ mg
C)   1200 lb. horse; dosage range 5–10 mg/kg
       minimum dose = _____ mg, maximum dose = _____ mg
D)   0.23 kg rat; dosage range 0.15–0.25 mg/g
       minimum dose = _____ mg, maximum dose = _____ mg
E)   1.7 kg bird; dosage range 2.2–4.4 mg/lb
       minimum dose = _____ mg, maximum dose = _____ mg

F) 300 kg gilt; dosage range 5–50 mg/lb
minimum dose = _____ mg, maximum dose = _____ mg

G) 1200 lb dairy cow; dosage range 5–8 mg/lb
minimum dose = _____ mg, maximum dose = _____ mg

4 Given the body weight, dosage, and tablet strength, determine how many tablets are needed per dose. Tablets may not be broken into anything smaller than a one-half tablet (i.e. no quarter tablets).

A) 67 lb dog; dosage is 10 mg/kg, 200 mg tablet _____ tablets per dose
B) 3.8 kg cat; dosage is 5 mg/lb, 10 mg tablet _____ tablets per dose
C) 900 lb horse; dosage is 1 mg/kg, 250 mg tablet _____ tablets per dose
D) 1.1 kg guinea pig; dosage is 10 mg/lb, 20 mg tablet _____ tablets per dose
E) 25.5 kg dog; dosage is 20 mg/lb, 350 mg tablet _____ tablets per dose
F) 6.25 lb cat; dosage is 15 mg/kg, 50 mg tablet _____ tablets per dose
G) 450 kg horse; dosage is 15 mg/lb, 5 g tablet _____ tablets per dose
H) 0.8 lb rat; dosage is 0.325 mg/lb, 0.5 mg tablet _____ tablets per dose

5 Given the body weight, dosage, and concentration of drug within the bottle, determine the volume of liquid needed per dose. Round to nearest 1/10 mL.

A) 48 lb dog; dosage is 25 mg/kg, bottle concentration 250 mg/mL _____ mL/dose
B) 4.2 kg cat; dosage is 20 mg/lb, bottle concentration 30 mg/mL _____ mL/dose
C) 1000 lb horse; dosage is 2.5 mg/kg, bottle concentration 400 mg/mL _____ mL/dose
D) 3 kg rabbit; dosage is 10 mg/lb, bottle concentration 15 mg/mL _____ mL/dose
E) 24 kg dog; dosage is 50 mg/lb, bottle concentration 500 mg/mL _____ mL/dose
F) 9.75 lb cat; dosage is 20 mg/kg, bottle concentration 75 mg/mL _____ mL/dose
G) 400 kg dairy cow; dosage is 10 mg/lb, bottle concentration 1.5 g/mL _____ mL/dose
H) 20 g mouse; dosage is 150 mg/kg, bottle concentration 12.5 mg/mL _____ mL/dose

6 Given the body weight, dosage, and concentration of drug listed as a percent, determine the volume of liquid needed per dose. Round to nearest 1/10 mL.

A) 22 lb dog, dosage is 50 mg/kg, 25% solution _____ mL/dose
B) 765 lb heifer, dosage is 10 mg/kg, 50% solution _____ mL/dose
C) 4.5 kg cat, dosage is 10 mg/lb, 2% solution _____ mL/dose
D) 16 kg dog, dosage is 20 mg/lb, 20% solution _____ mL/dose
E) 265 lb sow, dosage is 7.50 mg/kg, 42.5% solution _____ mL/dose

7 Given the body weight, dosage regimen, and tablet strength, determine the total number of tablets dispensed. Tablets can be broken into nothing smaller than a one-half tablet.

A) 110 lb dog; dosage regimen is 5 mg/kg q8h 10d PO, 250 mg tablets _____ tablets
B) 4.7 kg cat; dosage regimen is 20 mg/lb b.i.d. 5d PO, 100 mg tablets _____ tablets
C) 600 lb cow, dosage regimen is 10 mg/kg s.i.d. 10d PO, 3 g tablets _____ tablets
D) 38 kg dog, dosage regimen is 2 mg/lb q6h 12d PO, 200 mg tablets _____ tablets
E) 9 lb cat, dosage regimen is 50 mg/kg b.i.d. 5d PO, 100 mg tablets _____ tablets
F) 490 kg stallion, dosage regimen is 3 mg/lb q12h 7d, 800 mg tablets _____ tablets
G) 12.4 kg dog, dosage regimen is 6.8 mg/lb q6h 5d, 75 mg tablets _____ tablets
H) 47 lb dog, dosage regimen is 2 mg/kg s.i.d. 180d, 1/2 gr tablets _____ tablets

8 Look at Figures 8.5–8.10. For each of these syringes, indicate the volume of medication the syringe contains:

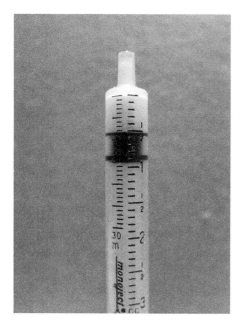

Figure 8.5

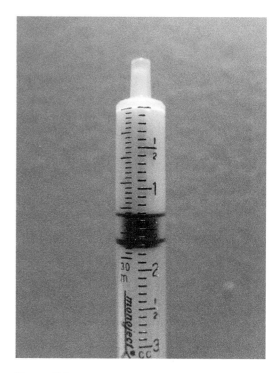

Figure 8.6

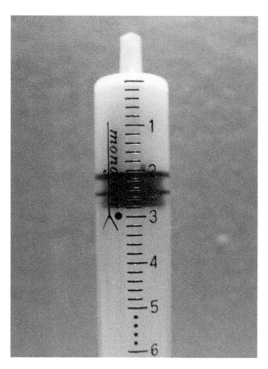

Figure 8.7

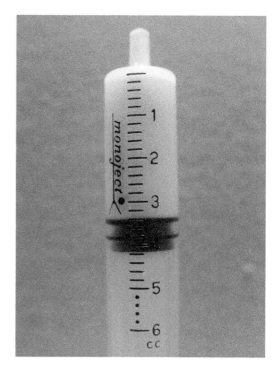

Figure 8.8

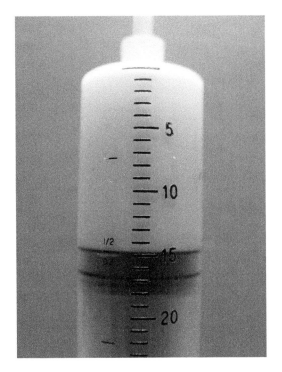

Figure 8.9   Figure 8.10

9   A veterinarian wants to use amikacin sulfate injectable in a 125 lb neonatal foal with pneumonia. Although the drug is not FDA approved for use in horses for this purpose, its use is allowable under the extra-label use guidelines as long as the horse is not to be used for human food. The recommended dosage range is 20–25 mg/kg IV or IM once daily. The drug is packaged in 48 mL vials at the concentration of 250 mg/mL. One vial costs $267.00. Given this information, answer the following questions.

A) What is the minimum and maximum milligram dose (to nearest 0.1 mg) this foal could have?
B) What is the volume of drug (to the nearest 0.1 mL) needed to deliver the minimum and the maximum dose?
C) If the entire 48 mL vial costs $267, how much does each mL cost (dollars per mL)?
D) How much does each minimum dose and each maximum dose cost?
E) Because the drug is given once daily, how many days can one vial provide a full minimum dose and a full maximum dose?

10 "Jacquie" the miniature poodle has a skin infection that needs to be treated with cefpodoxime antibiotic, shown in Figure 8.11. "Jocko," the terrier mix that lives with Jacquie, has a similar infection and will be treated with the same drug. The canine dosage is 5–10 mg/kg PO q24h. Jacquie weighs 13 lb and Jocko weighs 38 lb. The dogs need to be on the medication for 10 days. The 100 mg tablets cost the client $1.89 each and there is a $5.00 dispensing fee per drug order for any medication dispensed from the veterinary pharmacy (so Jacquie and Jocko *each* have a $5.00 dispensing fee in addition to the cost of the medication).

A) What is the minimum and maximum dose in milligrams (to nearest 0.1 mg) for Jacquie and Jocko?
B) Remembering that no tablet dose should be split into anything smaller than a half, what dose in tablets should Jacquie and Jocko each get? Remember also that with a dosage range, you should not have to go outside of that range to find the number of tablets that can be administered per dose.
C) Remembering the dispensing fee, what would be the total cost of the medications for Jacquie and Jocko to cover the full dosage regimen?

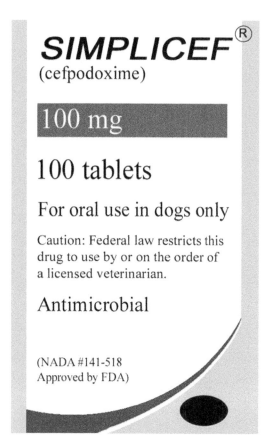

Figure 8.11

11 Mrs. Jones is going to be traveling with her three dogs in a motor home. She wants to get some ace-promazine tranquilizer for the animals since they are nervous travelers. The veterinary hospital carries only the 25 mg acepromazine tablets. These tablets are coated with a hard, smooth surface to facilitate swallowing, but which also makes them difficult to be split evenly into halves, requiring this dose form being dispensed as full tablets. Mrs. Jones' dogs weigh 30, 45, and 85 lb. The canine dose for this drug is a dose range of 0.55–2.2 mg/kg PO PRN. All doses selected for each animal should fit within the specified dose range.

A) What would be the minimum and maximum dose (in milligrams) for each dog, based upon the dosage range?
B) How many full tablets will be required to administer one dose for each of the three dogs?
C) Mrs. Jones' travel will require her giving the dogs four doses to each of the dogs. Provide Mrs. Jones enough tablets to provide the maximum dose for each dog in case she needs it. If the tablets sell for $0.75 each plus a dispensing fee of $8.00 per animal, what would be the total cost to Mrs. Jones for the three dogs?

9

Intravenous Infusion Calculations

OBJECTIVES

The student will be able to:

1) determine the flow rate for an IV infusion in milliliters given the drip rate and the calibration of an IV set,
2) determine the volume of IV fluid delivered given the flow rate and the time the infusion has been running,
3) determine the drip rate needed to deliver a known volume of fluid within a set period of time,
4) determine the required drip rate for administering drugs in IV fluids over a set time,
5) determine the drip rate to deliver IV maintenance fluid for dogs and cats, and
6) determine the appropriate stop time for administration of IV fluids based upon fluid volume to be administered and the rate of administration.

Drugs and intravenous fluids are often administered over a specific length of time and at a particular rate to ensure that the drug achieves and maintains the therapeutic concentrations needed to produce the beneficial effect while avoiding unnecessarily high peak concentrations that would produce toxic reactions or side effects. Because this balance of rate and time are critical to delivering the drug or IV fluids in an appropriate manner, the veterinary professional needs to thoroughly understand how to calculate infusion rates for medications and IV fluids.

9.1   Performing IV Infusions and the Use of IV Administration Sets

Drug orders may prescribe administering an intravenous drug either by infusion (drug "dripped" into the patient over time) or by a bolus (drug administered quickly in a "push"). Drug orders prescribing IV infusions describe the amount of drug to be administered, the route of administration, plus a time factor for administration. For example, a drug infusion may require "35 mg given intravenously over 5 minutes" or "250 mL of the 10 mg/mL concentration administered IV over 2 hours." The concepts of dosing and concentration covered in previous chapters will be applied to determine the correct amount of drug to be delivered via the IV infusion or bolus route of administration.

One of the factors used to determine how to deliver the correct amount of drug in the required time period is the IV equipment itself. IV fluids are administered via a gravity-driven IV administration set (tubing and attachments) or via an IV infusion pump. Syringe pumps may also be used to deliver relatively small volumes of drug automatically into an IV line. As the IV infusion pump and syringe pump provide for largely automated control over the IV fluid or drug administration rate, the discussion in this section will focus on using the gravity IV administration set (Figure 9.1).

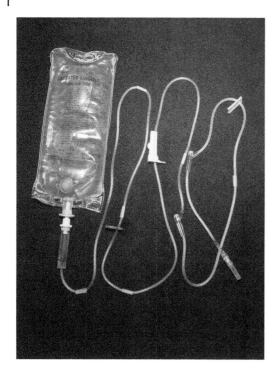

Figure 9.1 Intravenous fluid set – complete

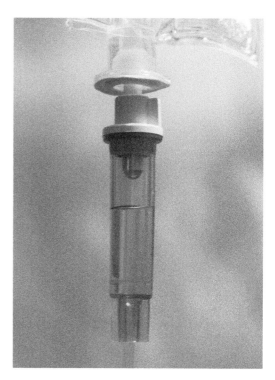

Figure 9.2 Drip chamber

A standard IV administration set includes intravenous tubing with a *spike* for inserting the IV tubing into an intravenous fluid bag or bottle on one end, and a *hub* that attaches the IV tubing to a needle or catheter at the other end. Just below the point where the spike attaches the tubing to the fluid bag or bottle is a clear plastic chamber called the *drip chamber* (Figure 9.2) through which the drops of fluid or drug can be observed as they pass from the fluid bag/bottle into the IV tubing. The rate at which drops pass through the drip chamber indicates the flow rate of IV fluids into the patient.

The intravenous tubing itself usually has either, or both, a *roller clamp* (Figure 9.3) or a *slide/occlusion clamp* (Figure 9.4) to regulate the flow of fluid through the IV tubing. An *injection port* (Figure 9.5) may also be incorporated into the IV tubing for injecting drugs into the flowing IV fluids. The injection port most commonly consists of a "Y"-shaped plastic tube with a rubber stopper on one of the branches of the "Y" through which medication can be injected. "T" ports are also available. A *burette* (a generic name) or *buretrol* (a trade name Buretrol® is often loosely applied to all burettes) is an additional calibrated chamber that is sometimes inserted into the IV line to allow a limited amount of drug or IV fluid to be slowly infused into the main line of the IV set.

9.2   The Basics of Setting IV Fluid Rate Using the Drip Chamber

As mentioned in Section 9.1, the rate at which IV fluid, with or without drug, is entering the patient is observed by counting the number of drops that pass through the drip chamber in a set amount of time (e.g. observing 5 drips per 10 seconds may be equivalent to 1 mL of fluid delivered to the patient every 40 seconds). To be able to accurately observe the IV fluid dripping from the bag/bottle through the drip chamber, the drip chamber must be only half filled with fluid when setting up the IV line. Filling the chamber all the way would prevent any drips from being observed, and not filling the chamber with any fluid may allow air in the chamber to flow along with the IV fluids into the patient. To half fill the drip chamber, hang

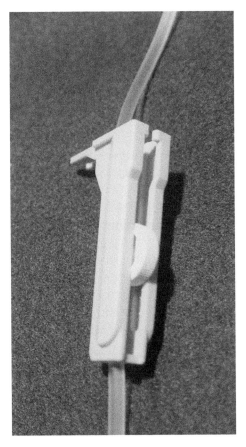

Figure 9.3 Roller clamp

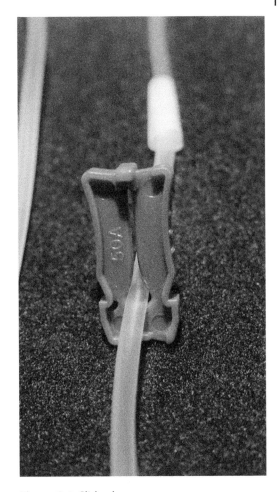

Figure 9.4 Slide clamp

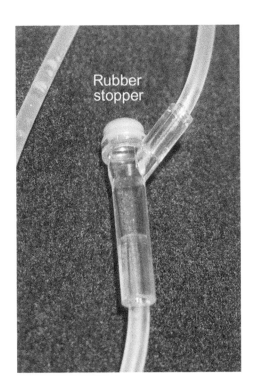

Figure 9.5 Injection port

the bag/bottle from an IV stand with the drip chamber below the bag/bottle, then squeeze the drip chamber slightly to expel some of the air from the drip chamber into the IV bag or bottle. Relax the squeeze and the drip chamber will partially fill with liquid.

To start the fluid flowing through the IV line, the slide clamp is moved or the wheel on the roller clamp rolled. Once the clamp is opened, drips can be observed dropping from the fluid bag/bottle into the liquid in the drip chamber. Rolling the clamp wheel or repositioning the slide clamp on the IV line will increase or decrease the flow rate.

The volume of fluid being delivered via an IV administration set is calculated by:

1) observing the rate of drips dropping through the drip chamber (drips per unit of time), and
2) the calibration of the IV administration set (number of drips that equal 1 mL).

The drip/mL calibration is usually listed on the package material that contains the IV administration set.

The most common forms of the "standard" or "macro drip" IV administration sets are calibrated so that 10, 15, or 20 drops equal 1 mL of fluid. The "micro drip" IV sets (sometimes referred to as "mini" or "pediatric" drip sets) are usually calibrated as 60 drops equals 1 mL. Remember that drops or drips are abbreviated as "gtt," which is the Latin abbreviation for "*guttae*" or drops. Therefore, the calibration listed on the package may appear as "20 gtt/mL" or "60 gtt/mL."

Here is an example to illustrate how the volume of IV fluid administered can be determined. A veterinary technician has obtained an IV set and has identified from the IV set box or container that this particular set is a standard or "macro drip" IV set calibrated so that 10 drops passing through the drip chamber equals 1 mL (10 gtt/mL). Once the IV set has been inserted into the fluids, the drip chamber correctly half filled, and the IV line hub inserted into the needle or catheter, the veterinary technician opens the roller clamp and drops start to fall through the chamber at the rate of 40 drops each minute. To determine the volume of IV fluid administered in that minute, the calibrated drip rate needs to be converted into the number of milliliters.

This problem is set up using the cancel-out method. The unknown X (what we want to find out) is the number of milliliters of IV fluid passed in 1 minute. The known value for the equation is the counted drips (gtt) passing through the drip chamber in 1 minute, and the conversion factor is the drip per milliliter (gtt/mL) calibration of the IV administration set:

$$\text{unknown } X \text{ unit} = \text{known value unit} \times \frac{\text{conversion factor with same units as unknown } X}{\text{conversion factor with same units as known value}}$$

$$X \text{ mL in 1 minute} = 40 \text{ gtt in 1 minute} \times \frac{1 \text{ mL}}{10 \text{ gtt}}$$

Notice how the equation is set up so that the unit "gtt" in the numerator would be canceled out by the "gtt" in the denominator, leaving only the units of milliliters (which is the unit of measurement for the answer in this problem).

$$X \text{ mL} = 40 \text{ gtt} \times \frac{1 \text{ mL}}{10 \text{ gtt}}$$

$$X \text{ mL} = 40 \,\cancel{\text{gtt}} \times \frac{1 \text{ mL}}{10 \,\cancel{\text{gtt}}}$$

$$X \text{ mL} = 40 \times \frac{1 \text{ mL}}{10}$$

$$X \text{ mL} = \frac{40 \text{ mL}}{10}$$

$$X \text{ mL} = 4 \text{ mL}$$

Therefore, seeing 40 drops passing through this drip chamber translates into 4 mL of fluid delivered to the patient for this particular IV set. Had the drip chamber had a 15 gtt equal to 1 mL calibration, the volume of fluid administered would have been 2.7 mL; and if a pediatric or micro drip chamber with 60 gtt equal to 1 mL calibration had been used the volume delivered would have only been 0.67 mL. Pediatric/micro drip sets allow a more precise fluid delivery rate to be set than the macro drip chamber IV sets.

In the previous problem, the veterinary technician observed the drip chamber for an entire minute to determine the drip rate. However, veterinary technicians are usually busy and they don't want to count drips for a whole minute to determine the rate, make an adjustment to the rate, and then count another minute to see if the adjustment is correct. Therefore, the drip rate is observed for a shorter period of time (e.g. 15 seconds) and the fluid flow rate of milliliters per minute is calculated from this. To do this, the unit of time must be factored into both sides of the original equation used above.

For example, if a veterinary technician observed 30 drips passing through the drip chamber in 15 seconds using an IV administration set calibrated to 10 drops/mL, how many mL would be delivered to the patient each minute?

The unknown X in this case is the milliliters of IV fluid delivered per minute; the known value is the 30 drips observed in 15 seconds, and the conversion factor that translates drips into milliliters is the IV set calibration of 10 drops equals 1 mL (10 drops/mL or 10 gtt/mL).

$$\text{unknown } X \text{ unit} = \text{known value unit} \times \frac{\text{conversion factor with same units as unknown } X}{\text{conversion factor with same units as known value}}$$

$$\frac{X\,\text{mL}}{\text{unit of time}} = \frac{\text{drips (gtt)}}{\text{unit of time}} \times \frac{1\,\text{mL}}{\text{drips equal to 1 mL for IV set}}$$

$$\frac{X\,\text{mL}}{\text{minute}} = \frac{30\,\text{drips (gtt)}}{15\,\text{seconds}} \times \frac{1\,\text{mL}}{10\,\text{drips}}$$

Note, however, that the time units are not the same on both sides of the equation, as there are minutes on the left and seconds on the right. Because the answer requires milliliters per minute, the 15 seconds must be converted to the equivalent minute fraction. To make the time units the same, a conversion factor can be added to the right side of the equation to convert seconds to minutes and, using the cancel-out method, the calculation should yield an answer in milliliters per minute.

$$\frac{X\,\text{mL}}{\text{minute}} = \frac{30\,\text{drips}}{15\,\text{seconds}} \times \frac{1\,\text{mL}}{10\,\text{drips}}$$

$$\frac{X\,\text{mL}}{\text{minute}} = \frac{30\,\text{drips}}{15\,\text{seconds}} \times \frac{60\,\text{seconds}}{1\,\text{minute}} \times \frac{1\,\text{mL}}{10\,\text{drips}}$$

$$\frac{X\,\text{mL}}{\text{minute}} = \frac{30\,\cancel{\text{drips}}}{15\,\text{seconds}} \times \frac{60\,\text{seconds}}{1\,\text{minute}} \times \frac{1\,\text{mL}}{10\,\cancel{\text{drips}}}$$

$$\frac{X\,\text{mL}}{\text{minute}} = \frac{30}{15\,\cancel{\text{seconds}}} \times \frac{60\,\cancel{\text{seconds}}}{1\,\text{minute}} \times \frac{1\,\text{mL}}{10}$$

$$\frac{X\,\text{mL}}{\text{minute}} = \frac{30}{15} \times \frac{60}{1\,\text{minute}} \times \frac{1\,\text{mL}}{10}$$

The units all cancel out appropriately, leaving only mL in the numerator (top part of the fraction) and minutes in the denominator (bottom part of the fraction) and so the answer is given in milliliters per minute.

$$\frac{X\,\text{mL}}{\text{minute}} = \frac{30}{15} \times \frac{60}{1\,\text{minute}} \times \frac{1\,\text{mL}}{10}$$

$$\frac{X\,\text{mL}}{\text{minute}} = \frac{30 \times 60 \times 1\,\text{mL}}{15 \times 1\,\text{minute} \times 10}$$

$$\frac{X\,\text{mL}}{\text{minute}} = \frac{1800\,\text{mL}}{150\,\text{minutes}}$$

$$\frac{X\,\text{mL}}{\text{minute}} = \frac{12\,\text{mL}}{\text{minute}}$$

Note that the longer the number of drips are observed, the more accurate assessment of the flow rate. For example, calculating the flow rate based upon the number of drips passing through the chamber in 30 seconds will provide a more accurate assessment of the fluid flow rate than counting drips for only 5 seconds. A 30 second count of 17 drips would be counted as either 2 or 3 drips if only measured for 5 seconds. The 5 second drip rate of 2 or 3 drips would extrapolate to between 24 and 36 drips per minute. In contrast. The 30 second observed rate of 17 drips would give a much more accurate drip rate of 34 drips per minute.

Once the drip rate is converted into a milliliter per minute flow rate, the volume of fluid delivered over any period of time can be determined by multiplying the number of minutes the rate has run by the milliliter per minute flow rate. For example, if the flow rate is 2 mL/min, then the volume of fluid delivered in 10 minutes would be calculated by multiplying 2 mL/min by 10 minutes.

9.3 Setting the IV Fluid Rate: Constant Rate Infusions (CRI)

The problems above answered the question: "How much IV fluid was delivered in a minute?" However, in veterinary medicine fluids and larger volumes of IV drugs are meant to be administered over a set time at a constant flow rate described as a *constant rate infusion* or *CRI*. To properly set up a CRI, the veterinary technician must know how much fluid needs to be delivered in what period of time, then translate that information into an observable drip rate using the calibration of the IV set. For example, a veterinary technician has received fluid orders to deliver 300 mL of IV fluid to a patient in 1 hour using a macro IV drip set calibrated to 15 gtt/mL. What drip rate (number of drops passing through the drip chamber) in a gravity flow IV set calibrated to 15 gtt/mL will produce the correct CRI flow rate?

To answer that question the basic formula for the cancel-out method is used. The unknown X component of the formula is drips per unit of time. Minutes for the unit of time can be used initially for the calculation and can be changed to seconds if need be after the calculation is performed. The known value is the volume of fluid to be delivered over the time unit by which it must be delivered (300 mL/h). Because the answer (the unknown X) is drips per minute, the known value should be in the same time unit. Instead of 300 mL/h, the time is changed to 300 mL per 60 minutes. Finally, the conversion factor for converting milliliters to number of drips is the drip rate of the IV administration set (15 drips/mL or 15 gtt/mL).

The problem is set up so that most of the units cancel out, leaving drips over minutes. Unlike the previous problem, where the conversion factor was set up as "1 mL over drips", the conversion factor for this problem must be flipped to be "drips over 1 mL" so that the units properly cancel out. This illustrates why it is so important to always include the units in the equation as a check to see if the calculation is properly set up.

$$\text{unknown}\,X\,\text{unit} = \text{known value unit} \times \frac{\text{conversion factor with same units as unknown}\,X}{\text{conversion factor with same units as known value}}$$

$$\frac{X \text{ drips}}{\text{minute}} = \frac{300 \text{ mL}}{60 \text{ minutes}} \times \frac{15 \text{ drips}}{1 \text{ mL}}$$

$$\frac{X \text{ drips}}{\text{minute}} = \frac{300 \,\cancel{\text{mL}}}{60 \text{ minutes}} \times \frac{15 \text{ drips}}{1 \,\cancel{\text{mL}}}$$

$$\frac{X \text{ drips}}{\text{minute}} = \frac{300 \times 15 \text{ drips}}{60 \text{ minutes} \times 1}$$

$$\frac{X \text{ drips}}{\text{minute}} = \frac{4500 \text{ drips}}{60 \text{ minutes}}$$

$$\frac{X \text{ drips}}{\text{minute}} = \frac{75 \text{ drips}}{1 \text{ minute}}$$

Once the drip rate is adjusted so 75 drops pass through the drip chamber each minute, the technician knows that 300 mL will be delivered in 1 hour. As stated previously, a technician would prefer not to wait the full minute to determine if the drip rate is correct, hence the drip rate expressed as drips per time in seconds allows for a quicker adjustment of the fluid rate. Converting the rate from drips per minute to drips per seconds uses the additional conversion factor of "1 minute equals 60 seconds" that was used in the previous problem. Again, it is important to include the units to determine if the calculation has been set up appropriately.

$$\frac{X \text{ drips}}{\text{second}} = \frac{75 \text{ drips}}{1 \text{ minute}} \times \frac{1 \text{ minute}}{60 \text{ seconds}}$$

$$\frac{X \text{ drips}}{\text{second}} = \frac{75 \text{ drips}}{1 \,\cancel{\text{minute}}} \times \frac{1 \,\cancel{\text{minute}}}{60 \text{ seconds}}$$

$$\frac{X \text{ drips}}{\text{second}} = \frac{75 \text{ drips}}{60 \text{ seconds}}$$

$$\frac{X \text{ drips}}{\text{second}} = \frac{1.25 \text{ drips}}{\text{second}}$$

It is impossible to determine if 0.25 drips (which equals 25/100 or a quarter of a drip) have passed through the drip chamber, therefore the drip rate per second must be converted to the nearest *whole* drips that would have to pass through the chamber. Mathematically to convert the fraction of a drip to a whole number of drips per seconds, the top and bottom of the equation must be multiplied by the same number. The veterinary technician might be able to "eyeball" the fraction to determine what number the fraction of drips can be multiplied by to create a whole number (e.g. 0.25 in the fraction multiplied by 4 would give the whole number 1).

$$\frac{1.25 \text{ drips}}{\text{second}} \times \frac{4}{4} = \frac{5 \text{ drips}}{4 \text{ seconds}}$$

If the appropriate conversion number is not readily apparent, then using 5, 10, 15, and 20 second intervals usually yields a drip number close to a whole number. For example, if the initial calculation yielded a drip rate of 0.467 drips per second, converting the answer to drips per 5, 10, 15, and 20 seconds gives a drip number that is close to a whole number.

$$\frac{0.467\,\text{drips}}{\text{second}} \times \frac{5}{5} = \frac{2.335\,\text{drips}}{5\,\text{seconds}}$$

$$\frac{0.467\,\text{drips}}{\text{second}} \times \frac{10}{10} = \frac{4.67\,\text{drips}}{10\,\text{seconds}}$$

$$\frac{0.467\,\text{drips}}{\text{second}} \times \frac{15}{15} = \frac{7.005\,\text{drips}}{15\,\text{seconds}}$$

$$\frac{0.467\,\text{drips}}{\text{second}} \times \frac{20}{20} = \frac{9.34\,\text{drips}}{20\,\text{seconds}}$$

Setting the IV fluid drip rate to 7 drips in 15 seconds would give the desired IV flow rate and be a manageable drip rate for the technician to monitor.

Had the initial time period to infuse the IV fluids been ordered for something other than 1 hour, the denominator of the 300 mL/h fraction would have been changed to reflect this time frame. The examples below show how the problem would have looked for fluid orders of 300 mL to be delivered over 2 hours (120 minutes), over 10 hours (600 minutes), and over 30 minutes (0.5 hour).

$$\frac{X\,\text{drips}}{\text{minute}} = \frac{300\,\text{mL}}{120\,\text{minutes}} \times \frac{15\,\text{drips}}{1\,\text{mL}}$$

$$\frac{X\,\text{drips}}{\text{minute}} = \frac{300\,\text{mL}}{600\,\text{minutes}} \times \frac{15\,\text{drips}}{1\,\text{mL}}$$

$$\frac{X\,\text{drips}}{\text{minute}} = \frac{300\,\text{mL}}{30\,\text{minutes}} \times \frac{15\,\text{drips}}{1\,\text{mL}}$$

To summarize how to set the fluid rate for X amount of volume delivered in Y amount of time:

1) set all time units to minutes,
2) use the required X volume/Y time (in minutes) as the known value,
3) use the calibrated drip rate of the IV administration set as the conversion factor,
4) once the drip rate per minute is calculated, convert it into seconds and find the most convenient set of seconds to count the drips passing through the drip chamber.

9.4 Calculating Infusion Rates when Adding Drugs to IV Fluids

Often drugs are added to the intravenous fluids as a means of infusing the drug dose over a set period of time. The method for determining the flow rate for the IV drug infusion uses the same principles used for determining the rate for IV fluids. An additional step involves determining the volume of drug that is to be added to the volume of IV fluids and then calculating the total amount of fluid to be delivered.

This can be best illustrated with an example. An animal needs 25 mg of drug to be infused over 4 hours. The concentration of drug in the vial is 10 mg/mL. The required dose of drug is going to be added to a 500 mL IV fluid bag for infusion over the 4 hours. The IV administration set has a calibrated drip rate of 20 gtt/mL. What drip rate is going to be needed to deliver the drug in 4 hours?

Although this may seem like a lot of information to put into an equation at one time, it becomes much more manageable when the equation is constructed one piece at a time using the principles shown in the previous problem. The first step is to determine the volume of drug to be administered that will deliver the required dose of 25 mg. This is the same calculation process as that discussed in Chapter 8 to determine the volume of liquid required to inject the prescribed mass (mg) of drug into a patient. The unknown X is the volume of liquid that must be withdrawn from the vial, the known value is the 25 mg dose, and the conversion factor to get from milligrams to milliliters is the concentration of the drug in the vial (10 mg/mL).

$$\text{unknown } X \text{ unit} = \text{known value unit} \times \frac{\text{conversion factor with same units as unknown } X}{\text{conversion factor with same units as known value}}$$

$$X \, \text{mL} = 25 \, \cancel{\text{mg}} \times \frac{1 \, \text{mL}}{10 \, \cancel{\text{mg}}}$$

$$X \, \text{mL} = \frac{25 \times 1 \, \text{mL}}{10}$$

$$X \, \text{mL} = 2.5 \, \text{mL}$$

2.5 mL of the drug must be added to the 500 mL IV fluid bag to deliver the 25 mg of drug the patient needs. The total volume in the IV fluid bag is therefore 502.5 mL. Some clinicians choose not to calculate the combined volume of drug and fluids to determine the fluid administration rate because the volume added by the drug is negligible. However, it is a better practice to always include the volume of drug so that when larger volume of drugs, especially toxic drugs like cancer chemotherapeutic drugs, are delivered the most accurate drip rate will be mathematically determined. For this problem, 502.5 mL of drug plus IV fluids must be delivered in 4 hours. The next step is to determine the required rate of delivery using the cancel-out method, as was described in Section 9.3.

$$\text{unknown } X \text{ unit} = \text{known value unit} \times \frac{\text{conversion factor with same units as unknown } X}{\text{conversion factor with same units as known value}}$$

The unknown X is the rate in drips per minute (or drips per several seconds), the known value is the 502.5 mL in 4 hours (expressed as 502.5 mL over 4 hours), and the conversion factor for converting the known into the unknown X drips per time is the calibration of the IV set drip rate of 10 drips equals 1 mL (10 drips/mL or 10 gtt/mL).

$$\frac{X \, \text{drips}}{\text{minute}} = \frac{502.5 \, \text{mL}}{4 \, \text{hours}} \times \frac{10 \, \text{drips}}{1 \, \text{mL}}$$

As was emphasized in previous examples, the time units on either side of the equation need to be the same. The veterinary technician can either convert the 4 hours into the equivalent number of minutes in their head, or an additional conversion factor can be added to convert hours to minutes (60 minutes equals 1 hour).

$$\frac{X \, \text{drips}}{\text{minute}} = \frac{502.5 \, \text{mL}}{4 \, \text{hours}} \times \frac{1 \, \text{hour}}{60 \, \text{minutes}} \times \frac{10 \, \text{drips}}{1 \, \text{mL}}$$

As before, the unknown X time factor can be set initially to minutes but will eventually be converted to drips per some set of seconds after the initial calculation. A quick review of the equation verifies that most of the units on the right of the equation will cancel out, leaving only drips in the numerator and minutes in the denominator, which is the same arrangement as the unknown X units on the left of the equal sign.

$$\frac{X\,\text{drips}}{\text{minute}} = \frac{502.5\,\cancel{\text{mL}}}{4\,\text{hours}} \times \frac{1\,\text{hour}}{60\,\text{minutes}} \times \frac{10\,\text{drips}}{1\,\cancel{\text{mL}}}$$

$$\frac{X\,\text{drips}}{\text{minute}} = \frac{502.5}{4\,\cancel{\text{hours}}} \times \frac{1\,\cancel{\text{hour}}}{60\,\text{minutes}} \times \frac{10\,\text{drips}}{1}$$

$$\frac{X\,\text{drips}}{\text{minute}} = \frac{502.5}{4} \times \frac{1}{60\,\text{minutes}} \times \frac{10\,\text{drips}}{1}$$

The equation can now be calculated to give drips per minute needed to deliver 502.5 mL in 4 hours.

$$\frac{X\,\text{drips}}{\text{minute}} = \frac{502.5 \times 1 \times 10\,\text{drips}}{4 \times 60\,\text{minutes} \times 1}$$

$$\frac{X\,\text{drips}}{\text{minute}} = \frac{5025\,\text{drips}}{240\,\text{minutes}}$$

The number of drips per second can then be determined using the conversion of 1 minute equals 60 seconds.

$$\frac{X\,\text{drips}}{\text{second}} = \frac{5025\,\text{drips}}{240\,\text{minutes}} \times \frac{1\,\text{minute}}{60\,\text{seconds}}$$

$$\frac{X\,\text{drips}}{\text{second}} = \frac{5025\,\text{drips}}{240\,\cancel{\text{minutes}}} \times \frac{1\,\cancel{\text{minute}}}{60\,\text{seconds}}$$

$$\frac{X\,\text{drips}}{\text{second}} = \frac{0.349\,\text{drips}}{\text{second}}$$

The conversion factor for minutes converted to seconds could have also been performed within the initial calculation, saving this additional step. As discussed in the previous section, a fraction of a second is not useful for determining a drip rate, so the drip rate can be mathematically converted into equivalent drips per 5, 10, 15, or 20 seconds to find a more useful rate.

$$\frac{0.349\,\text{drips}}{\text{second}} \times \frac{5}{5} = \frac{1.745\,\text{drips}}{5\,\text{seconds}}$$

$$\frac{0.349\,\text{drips}}{\text{second}} \times \frac{10}{10} = \frac{3.49\,\text{drips}}{10\,\text{seconds}}$$

$$\frac{0.349\,\text{drips}}{\text{second}} \times \frac{15}{15} = \frac{5.235\,\text{drips}}{15\,\text{seconds}}$$

$$\frac{0.349\,\text{drips}}{\text{second}} \times \frac{20}{20} = \frac{6.98\,\text{drips}}{20\,\text{seconds}}$$

By rounding to the nearest whole second, the veterinary technician can adjust the drip rate to either 5 drips in 15 seconds or 7 drips in 20 seconds, delivering the desired amount of the fluid plus drug in the required 4 hour period of time.

To summarize, when calculating a drip rate for infusion of a drug in IV fluids within a set period of time, the steps would be:

1) determine the *volume* of drug needed to be added to the IV fluid to deliver the dose,
2) determine the total volume of IV fluid and drug to be delivered in the set time frame, and
3) determine the drip rate in drips per some number of seconds to deliver the total fluid.

9.5 Calculating Standard IV Fluid Rates

There are standard rates of IV fluid administration used in specific clinical circumstances, such as to replace normal fluid loss in an animal that is not drinking or eating, or to counter the hypotensive effects of shock. The veterinary professional should know how to utilize these standard rates and should be able to calculate them quickly and accurately as they are often used under emergency circumstances.

Formulas for IV fluid rates used in human and veterinary medicine are based upon mathematical and biological models and should provide directions for how much fluid the body needs. These formulas take advantage of a unique relationship that exists between the weight (mass) of water and its corresponding volume. Normally mass (weight) and volume are two separate measuring systems that don't have a consistent mathematical relationship between units of mass and units of volume. Difference substances have different densities and therefore 1 cubic centimeter (cc) or 1 mL of one substance won't weigh the same amount as 1 mL of another substance. For example, 1 cc of a liquid metal such as mercury would have a different mass (weight) than the same volume of another liquid, say 1 cc of cooking oil. Thus 1 kg of substance X would not have the same volume as 1 kg of substance Y. The point here is that, with very few exceptions, medical math calculations cannot equate a given mass (weight) with a given volume.

The exception to this is water. In the late 1700s 1 kg of weight (mass) was defined as the weight of 1 L (volume) of water at the temperature of melting ice. Hence, by defining a unit of mass (weight) by a particular volume of water, a relationship was defined between mass and volume for water that is used in medicine today. 1 kg of water is equivalent to 1 L of water, therefore the density of water is 1 g/mL. The density of blood is very close to the density of water; blood is slightly denser, and therefore has slightly more mass per milliliter (the density of blood is 1.05 g/mL). Still, the similarity between blood and water in terms of density is close enough that if an animal has lost 1 kg (mass) of body weight due to blood loss from an injury, it can be assumed the animal needs 1 L (volume) of blood to restore its blood volume. The same is true for dehydration, where the body weight of the animal decreases because of a net loss of body water. In an animal that normally weighs 20 kg and has lost 1 kg of body weight due to body water loss (e.g. diarrhea and vomiting), it can be assumed that 1 L of IV fluids is needed to replace the lost body water. The key point is that the unique "kilogram mass to liter volume" relationship of water, and by extension blood, is often used medically in calculations used to determine the volume of IV fluids an animal should be administered.

Maintenance IV fluid rates are designed to provide the body with just enough IV fluids to replenish fluid lost via normal urination, evaporation, or metabolism. Different sources can cite slightly different rates, but the maintenance IV fluid rates shown below are the rates cited in the 2013 AAHA/AAFP (American Animal Hospital Association and the American Association of Feline Practitioners) Fluid Therapy Guidelines for Dogs and Cats:

    Dogs: 2–6 mL/kg/h
    Cats: 2–3 mL/kg/h

What volume of IV fluid *per hour* would a 15 kg dog that is not consuming food or water need to replace body water normally lost through urination, evaporation, or metabolism? Because the recommended maintenance fluid rate is listed as a range of 2–6 mL/kg body weight per hour, the minimum volume per hour and the maximum volume per hour must both be calculated.

Using the standard cancel-out formula, the unknown X is the number of milliliters needed per hour (the time unit for the answer is assumed to be 1 hour). The known value is the animal's weight in kilograms, and the conversion factor is the species volume per kilogram body weight (mL/kg).

$$\text{unknown}\,X\,(\text{minimum rate}) = 15\,\text{kg} \times \frac{2\,\text{mL}}{\text{kg}}$$

$$\text{unknown}\,X\,(\text{minimum rate}) = 15\,\cancel{\text{kg}} \times 2\,\text{mL}\cancel{\text{kg}}$$

$$\text{unknown}\,X = 30\,\text{mL per hour minimum}$$

$$\text{unknown}\,X\,(\text{maximum rate}) = 15\,\text{kg} \times \frac{6\,\text{mL}}{\text{kg}}$$

$$\text{unknown}\,X = 90\,\text{mL per hour maximum}$$

The calculation says that a 15 kg dog needs 30–90 mL of IV fluids per hour to maintain its hydration. Knowing this, the mL per hour can be converted to mL per minutes or mL per seconds, and finally to drips per set of seconds, as was done in the previous problems. If we were using a 15 gtt/mL calibrated IV drip set, the calculation for the minimum drip rate would look like this:

$$\frac{X\,\text{drips}}{\text{second}} = \frac{30\,\text{mL}}{1\,\text{hour}} \times \frac{1\,\text{hour}}{60\,\text{minutes}} \times \frac{1\,\text{minute}}{60\,\text{seconds}} \times \frac{15\,\text{drips}}{1\,\text{mL}}$$

$$\frac{X\,\text{drips}}{\text{second}} = \frac{30\,\cancel{\text{mL}}}{1\,\cancel{\text{hour}}} \times \frac{1\,\cancel{\text{hour}}}{60\,\cancel{\text{minutes}}} \times \frac{1\,\cancel{\text{minute}}}{60\,\text{seconds}} \times \frac{15\,\text{drips}}{1\,\cancel{\text{mL}}}$$

$$\frac{X\,\text{drips}}{\text{second}} = \frac{30 \times 1 \times 1 \times 15\,\text{drips}}{1 \times 60 \times 60\,\text{seconds} \times 1}$$

$$\frac{X\,\text{drips}}{\text{second}} = \frac{450\,\text{drips}}{3600\,\text{seconds}}$$

$$\frac{X\,\text{drips}}{\text{second}} = \frac{0.125\,\text{drips}}{\text{second}}$$

A fractional drip per second isn't usable, so the fractional drip must be converted to a whole drip per a number of seconds. By remembering the important fraction-to-decimal conversions from Table 3.4, the technician can recognize that the decimal 0.125 is equivalent to the fraction 1/8. To change the fractional drip to a whole drip only requires multiplying by its reciprocal 8 (1/8 × 8 = 1). So, if the minimum drip rate needed to deliver the appropriate amount of IV fluid for a 15 kg dog would is 1/8th of a drip per second, then multiplying both 0.125 drip and the time unit of 1 second by 8 gives a manageable drip rate of 1 drip every 8 seconds.

Because the IV maintenance fluid rate is a range of IV flow rates (2 to 6 mL/kg/h), the maximum drip rate would also have to be calculated. The same procedure used to calculate the minimum flow rate could be repeated to calculate the maximum flow rate; however, in this case it is much easier to see that the maximum drip rate (6 mL/kg/h) is mathematically 3× the minimum drip rate (2 mL/kg/h). Therefore, the maximum drip rate can be calculated simply by multiplying the minimum drip rate by 3. The acceptable IV maintenance fluid drip rate for a 15 kg dog is any drip rate between 1 and 3 drips per 8 seconds.

The 2013 AAHA/AAFP Fluid Therapy Guidelines describe another formula for calculating the daily (24 hour) volume of maintenance fluid in milliliters needed for dogs and cats:

Dogs: $132 \times (\text{body weight in kg})^{0.75}$
Cats: $80 \times (\text{body weight in kg})^{0.75}$

These formulas take into account a mathematical species factor expressed as 132 and 80 such that the only calculation that needs to be made is to multiply the species factor by the animal's weight raised to the 0.75 power or 0.75 exponent. Using the exponent is easy to do with a calculator using the x^y function where x is the animals weight in kilograms and y is 0.75. As an example, here is the calculation process used to determine the milliliters per day the 15 kg dog would need:

$$\frac{X \text{ mL fluid}}{\text{day}} = 132 \times 15^{0.75}$$

Note that the use of the 132 factor in this formula means that units on the right side of the equation don't have to be tracked or canceled out. This is simply a "plug-in and calculate" formula. The first step is to determine what value is represented by 15 raised to the 0.75 power. Using a calculator, input the value 15 first, then hit the x^y function button. Next put in 0.75 for the exponential part of the calculation. Pressing the equal sign will perform the calculation, giving the answer 7.622. These steps may vary slightly with other types of calculators, but essentially it is still the same process: put 15 in for the base x and put 0.75 in for the exponent y. The calculated value (7.622) is multiplied by the 132 factor to give the final number of mL that is needed to be administered in 24 hours or 1 day for this patient.

$$\frac{X \text{ mL}}{\text{day}} = 132 \times 7.622$$

$$\frac{X \text{ mL}}{\text{day}} = 1006$$

Giving 1006 mL (or a little more than a liter) of IV fluid per day should provide a 15 kg dog with enough fluids to maintain its normal hydration. In the previous maintenance IV fluid calculation where a range of flow rates was determined, the 15 kg dog needed 30–90 mL/h, which converts to 720–2160 mL in 24 hours. Thus, both calculation methods give similar answers (the 1006 mL/day is within the range of 720–2160 mL/day). The advantage of using the range of fluid rates calculation is that it offers the flexibility to adjust the flow rate within that calculated range of flow rates to compensate for conditions that might contribute to the patient losing more water than normal (e.g. polyuria from renal disease, diabetes mellitus, or greater evaporative loss into a dry environment with low humidity).

Often animals presented to the hospital needing maintenance IV fluid therapy are also dehydrated from water loss associated with disease or lack of water/food intake. While the maintenance IV fluid matches the continued loss of water through normal urination, evaporation, or metabolism, it does not replace the deficit of water caused by disease that is contributing to the dehydrated state. Therefore, dehydrated animals must receive additional IV fluid above the maintenance fluid volume to return the animal back to "normal" hydration status. To safely rehydrate an animal, sufficient IV fluid is given over several hours to correct the dehydration without overhydrating the animal (fluid overload) or increasing the fluid volume in the blood too quickly and placing unnecessary work load on the heart of patients with heart failure. The formula used to determine the volume of fluid needed to correct for dehydration is shown below:

$$\text{fluid volume to correct dehydration (L)} = \text{body weight (kg)} \times \%\text{dehydration (as a decimal)}$$

The percentage of body dehydration is estimated by physical examination of the skin turgor (how quickly the skin falls back in place when pulled up), wet/dry nose and mucous membranes, sunken eye, or thready pulse (weak, rapid pulse). Most clinical textbooks describe the physical characteristics that reflect percentages of dehydration. If the 15 kg dog used in the examples was also determined to be 8% dehydrated (classified as moderate dehydration), the body weight and the decimal number equivalent of 8% would be plugged into the formula to determine the amount of fluid needed to correct the dehydration.

$$\text{fluid volume to correct dehydration (L)} = 15 \times 0.08$$

$$\text{fluid volume to correct dehydration (L)} = 1.2\,\text{L}$$

This 15 kg dog needs 1.2 L of IV fluids to replace water lost by disease or lack of water intake. One of the most common mistakes made in doing this calculation is incorrectly converting the % value into the wrong decimal value. For example, 8% is sometimes incorrectly converted to 0.8 instead of the correct 0.08 (8% = 8/100 = 0.08). Failure to do this conversion properly can result in a fluid calculation that, if administered, could result in a potentially fatal fluid overload.

To determine the amount of fluid to be given in 24 hours to correct for dehydration and compensate for normal fluid loss, the maintenance IV fluid volume for 24 hours and the dehydration correction fluid volume must be added together. Previously it was determined that the 15 kg dog needed 720–2160 mL or 1006 mL (depending on method used to calculate) of fluid in 24 hours to replenish normal fluid loss. The clinician decided to order 1000 mL (1 L) of fluids for maintenance and 1.2 L of fluid (1200 mL) to correct the deficit. Total fluid to be delivered in 24 hours is 2.2 L or 2200 mL. The IV fluid set is calibrated at 10 drips/mL (10 gtt/mL). The equation for calculation the drip rate is set up in the same way as previous examples, but includes conversion factors for converting hours to seconds and for converting milliliters to drips.

$$\frac{X\,\text{drips}}{\text{second}} = \frac{2200\,\text{mL}}{24\,\text{hours}} \times \frac{1\,\text{hour}}{60\,\text{minutes}} \times \frac{1\,\text{minute}}{60\,\text{seconds}} \times \frac{10\,\text{drips}}{1\,\text{mL}}$$

$$\frac{X\,\text{drips}}{\text{second}} = \frac{2200\,\cancel{\text{mL}}}{24\,\cancel{\text{hours}}} \times \frac{1\,\cancel{\text{hour}}}{60\,\cancel{\text{minutes}}} \times \frac{1\,\cancel{\text{minute}}}{60\,\text{seconds}} \times \frac{10\,\text{drips}}{1\,\cancel{\text{mL}}}$$

$$\frac{X\,\text{drips}}{\text{second}} = \frac{2200 \times 1 \times 1 \times 10\,\text{drips}}{24 \times 60 \times 60\,\text{seconds} \times 1}$$

$$\frac{X\,\text{drips}}{\text{second}} = \frac{22\,000\,\text{drips}}{86\,400\,\text{seconds}}$$

$$\frac{X\,\text{drips}}{\text{second}} = \frac{0.2546\,\text{drips}}{\text{second}}$$

$$\frac{0.2546\,\text{drips}}{\text{second}} \times \frac{4}{4} = \frac{1.0184\,\text{drips}}{4\,\text{seconds}}$$

$$\frac{0.2546\,\text{drips}}{\text{second}} \times \frac{6}{6} = \frac{1.5276\,\text{drips}}{6\,\text{seconds}}$$

$$\frac{0.2546\,\text{drips}}{\text{second}} \times \frac{8}{8} = \frac{2.0368\,\text{drips}}{8\,\text{seconds}}$$

If the technician sets the drip rate to 1 drop every 4 seconds or 2 drops every 8 seconds, the required dehydration correction fluid volume and maintenance fluid will be delivered in 24 hours.

9.6 Calculating IV Fluid Rate Stop Times

Sometimes a IV fluid rate is determined for a patient (e.g. maintenance IV fluid rate for a cat at 2 mL/kg/h) but the rate is paired with a limit on the volume of fluid to be given (e.g. stop after administering 250 mL of a 1 L bag). It is important for the veterinary technician to be able to determine when to stop the flow rate if a fluid pump with a built-in volume calculator is not being used.

The rate of delivery can be calculated by the veterinary technician either using the calculations described previously in this chapter, or the veterinarian can order a rate based upon the condition of the animal (e.g. 2 × the maintenance fluid rate). Either way, once the rate has been determined, the time to deliver a set volume can be readily determined.

To illustrate this, a veterinarian ordered the 15 kg dog in the previous examples to have a maintenance IV fluid rate of 3 mL/kg/h with a limit of 500 mL of fluid from a 1000 mL fluid bag. The veterinary technician will need to calculate the rate for a 15 kg dog given the standard IV fluid rate of 3 mL/kg/h.

$$\text{number of mL in an hour} = 15\,\text{kg} \times \frac{3\,\text{mL}}{\text{kg}}$$

$$\text{number of mL in an hour} = 45\,\text{mL}$$

The flow rate needed to deliver maintenance fluid for a 15 kg dog is 45 mL/h. The amount of time needed to deliver 500 mL at the rate of 45 mL in an hour can be set up using the cancel-out method. The unknown X is the time in hours the fluid rate needs to run, the known value is the 500 mL that need to be delivered, and the conversion factor is the rate expressed mathematically as either 45 mL/h or 1 hour/45 mL.

$$\text{unknown}\,X\,\text{unit} = \text{known value unit} \times \frac{\text{conversion factor with same units as unknown}\,X}{\text{conversion factor with same units as known value}}$$

$$\text{time needed for IV infusion (hours)} = 500\,\text{mL} \times \frac{1\,\text{hour}}{45\,\text{mL}}$$

Notice how the rate in the conversion factor had to be arranged as 1 hour over 45 mL for the milliliters to cancel out, leaving just the time unit of hours in the numerator (top of the fraction). If the conversion factor had been set up as 45 mL/h, the calculation would have been incorrect.

$$\text{time needed for IV infusion (hours)} = 500\,\text{mL} \times \frac{1\,\text{hour}}{45\,\text{mL}}$$

$$\text{time needed for IV infusion (hours)} = \frac{500\,\text{hours}}{45}$$

$$\text{time needed for IV infusion (hours)} = 11.111\,\text{hours}$$

It is going to take a little over 11 hours for 500 mL of fluid to be administered to the patient. However, just like a fraction of a drip is not useful for determining rate, a fraction of an hour is usually not useful for determining the time elapsed or time needed. Therefore, the fractional 0.111 hour needs to be converted into minutes by using the 60 minutes/1 hour or 1 hour/60 minutes conversion factor.

$$\text{minutes} = 0.111\,\text{hour} \times \frac{60\,\text{minutes}}{1\,\text{hour}}$$

$$\text{minutes} = \frac{0.111 \times 60\,\text{minutes}}{1}$$

$$\text{minutes} = 6.66\,\text{minutes}$$

It is going to take 11 hours, 6 minutes (plus a little) to administer the 500 mL of fluid. But again, a fraction of a minute is not helpful, so the 0.66 fraction of minute can likewise be converted into seconds.

$$\text{seconds} = 0.66\,\text{minute} \times \frac{60\,\text{seconds}}{1\,\text{minute}}$$

$$\text{seconds} = \frac{0.66 \times 60\,\text{seconds}}{1}$$

$$\text{seconds} = 39.6\,\text{seconds, which rounds to 40 seconds}$$

Thus, it will take a total of 11 hours, 6 minutes, and 40 seconds to deliver 500 mL at the rate of 45 mL/h.

For practical reasons, infusions of this length are usually rounded to the nearest minute. So, a total infusion time that has 30 or more seconds would be rounded up to the next minute (e.g. 6 minutes 40 seconds would round up to 7 minutes), and an infusion of less than 30 seconds would simply be rounded to the same number of minutes (e.g. 6 minutes and 20 seconds would round to 6 minutes). In the example above, the infusion would run for 11 hours and 7 minutes.

Once the duration of the IV infusion has been determined, the veterinary technician needs to identify the "stop time" that will occur 11 hours, 6 minutes, and 40 seconds from the time the infusion began. Calculating the stop time in one's head can often be confusing, resulting in errors in stop times and subsequently more or less of the required volume of fluid being administered. Therefore, using a fairly simple stepwise method increases the odds that the timing will be correct. The technique will vary slightly if you are using a 12-hour clock (12 hours, a.m. and p.m.) or a 24-hour clock (from 0:00 to 24:00). The technique described here is for the 12-hour clock and for infusions lasting less than 24 hours.

- Step 1: Add the number of hours needed for the infusion to the hour the infusion will start (e.g. add to 3 hours if the start time is going to be 3:45 p.m.).

- Step 2: If the number of total hours is less than 12, record the number of hours and go onto Step 3. If the number of total hours if greater than 12, subtract 12 from the totaled hours and switch from the current a.m. to p.m. or from p.m. to a.m. for the answer and then go to Step 3.
- Step 3: Add the number of minutes needed for the infusion to the minutes the infusion will start (e.g. add to 45 minutes if the start time is going to be 3:45 p.m.).
- Step 4: If the number of total minutes is less than 60, record the number and go onto Step 5. If the number is greater than 60, subtract 60 from the totaled minutes and add 1 hour to the number of hours in Steps 1 and 2 and then go to Step 5.
- Step 5: The total number of hours and minutes from the calculation, with an appropriate switch of a.m. or p.m. as needed, is the stop time for the infusion.

The following example illustrates how this is done. In the previous example with the 15 kg dog needing a maintenance fluid rate for 11 hours and 7 minutes to deliver 250 mL of fluid, the veterinary technician is going to start the flow rate at 10:55 a.m.

- Step 1: 11 hours infusion time is added to 10 hours for the start time to give 21 hours total.
- Step 2: The number of hours is greater than 12 so 12 is subtracted from 21 to give 9 hours. The a.m. (from 10:55 a.m.) is changed to p.m.
- Step 3: 7 minutes infusion time is added to 55 minutes for the start time to give 62 minutes total.
- Step 4: The number of minutes is greater than 60 so 60 is subtracted from 62 to give 2 minutes. An additional hour is added to the hours to give 10 hours.
- Step 5: The stop time is 10:02 p.m. (10 hours, plus minutes, plus the switch from a.m. to p.m.).

Note: for safety purposes it is useful to indicate the DAY of the stop time, just to be clear. If the IV fluid infusion is started the afternoon of December 1st and ends at 3:05 a.m. on December 2nd, the stop time should include the date, "December 2." For infusions lasting more than 24 hours, Step 2 would have to be repeated, changing a.m. to p.m. (or p.m. to a.m.) each time until the number of hours is less than 12.

If the hospital runs on a 24-hour clock where 00:00 is midnight, 12:00 is noon, 18:00 is 6:00 p.m., and 23:59 is one minute before midnight, the process described above substitutes 24 hours for the 12 hours (subtract 24 hours if total hours exceeds 24) and indicate the date of the stop time (e.g. 21:45 December 2).

9.7 Chapter 9 Practice Problems

1   Given the observed drip rate and IV set calibrations (gtt/mL), determine the volume flow in milliliters per minute:

A) 10 gtt/mL, 20 drips/min = _____ mL/min
B) 15 gtt/mL, 300 drips/min = _____ mL/min
C) 20 gtt/mL, 320 drips/min = _____ mL/min
D) 60 gtt/mL, 1260 drips/min = _____ mL/min
E) 10 gtt/mL, 1 drip/s = _____ mL/min
F) 20 gtt/mL, 1 drip/s = _____ mL/min
G) 60 gtt/mL, 2 drips/s = _____ mL/min
H) 20 gtt/mL, 3 drips every 6 seconds = _____ mL/min
I)   15 gtt/mL, 15 drips every 10 seconds = _____ mL/min
J)   60 gtt/mL, 30 drips every 15 seconds = _____ mL/min

2   Given the IV set calibration, observed drip rate, and the length of time the IV fluid has run, determine the volume of fluid (in mL) delivered in the stated length of time:

A) IV set calibration = 10 gtt/mL, observed drip rate = 2 drips/second, for 15 minutes
B) IV set calibration = 20 gtt/mL, observed drip rate = 1 drips/second, for 10 minutes
C) IV set calibration = 60 gtt/mL, observed drip rate = 10 drips/20 seconds, for 20 minutes
D) IV set calibration = 15 gtt/mL, observed drip rate = 30 drips/45 seconds, for 15 minutes
E) IV set calibration = 20 gtt/mL, observed drip rate = 2 drips/5 seconds, for 12 minutes
F) IV set calibration = 60 gtt/mL, observed drip rate = 12 drips/5 seconds, for 30 minutes
G) IV set calibration = 15 gtt/mL, observed drip rate = 7 drips/10 seconds, for 40 minutes
H) IV set calibration = 20 gtt/mL, observed drip rate = 3 drips/15 seconds, for one hour
I) IV set calibration = 15 gtt/mL, observed drip rate = 22 drips/10 seconds, for 3.5 hours
J) IV set calibration = 60 gtt/mL, observed drip rate = 8 drips/5 seconds, for 12 hours

3   Given the volume of drug or fluid that needs to be administered, the time by which it needs to be administered, and the calibration of the IV drip set, determine the required drip rate in *X drips in Y seconds* needed to deliver the volume on time:

A) Volume needed = 810 mL, time to deliver = 6 hours, IV drip set calibration = 20 gtt/mL
B) Volume needed = 180 mL, time to deliver = 12 hours, IV drip set calibration = 60 gtt/mL
C) Volume needed = 768 mL, time to deliver = 4 hours, IV drip set calibration = 15 gtt/mL
D) Volume needed = 162 mL, time to deliver = 6 hours, IV drip set calibration = 20 gtt/mL
E) Volume needed = 0.9 L, time to deliver = 12 hours, IV drip set calibration = 60 gtt/mL
F) Volume needed = 4.5 L, time to deliver = 15 hours, IV drip set calibration = 20 gtt/mL
G) Volume needed = 120 mL, time to deliver = 0.5 hours, IV drip set calibration = 15 gtt/mL
H) Volume needed = 0.2 L, time to deliver = 10 hours, IV drip set calibration = 60 gtt/mL
I) Volume needed = 4 L, time to deliver = 10 hours, IV drip set calibration = 15 gtt/mL
J) Volume needed = 1.25 L, time to deliver = 15 hours, IV drip set calibration = 10 gtt/mL

4   Given the IV drug dose, the IV drug concentration, the volume of fluids into which the drug volume is going to be added, the amount of time ordered to infuse the combined volume of drug and IV fluid, and the calibration of the IV set; determine the drip rate in *X drips in Y seconds* needed to deliver the IV drug on time. Make the calculation using the total volume of fluid plus the volume of drug added to the fluid. Arrive at a drip rate that provides the most accurate delivery for drip rate that is 20 seconds or less (e.g. most accurate drip rate within the range of *X* drips per 1 second to *X* drips per 20 seconds).

A) 600 mg IV drug, 200 mg/mL concentration, 100 mL IV fluid, 4.25 hours, IV set calibration 20 gtt/mL
B) 250 mg IV drug, 25 mg/mL concentration, 1 L IV fluid, 12 hours, IV set calibration 10 gtt/mL
C) 4.8 g IV drug, 40 mg/mL concentration, 100 mL IV fluid, 5 and a half hours, IV set calibration 15 gtt/mL
D) 450 mg IV drug, 5 mg/mL concentration, ¼ liter, 4 hours, IV set calibration 20 gtt/mL
E) 220 mg IV drug, 12.5 mg/mL concentration, 750 mL IV fluid, 6 hours, IV set calibration 15 gtt/mL
F) 0.1 mg IV drug, 0.125 mg/mL concentration, 100 mL IV fluid, 2 hours, IV set calibration 60 gtt/mL
G) 350 mg IV drug, 25 mg/mL concentration, 1 L IV fluid, 12 hours, IV set calibration 60 gtt/mL
H) 48.5 mg IV drug, 10 mg/mL concentration, 300 mL IV fluid, 1½ hours, IV set calibration 15 gtt/mL
I) 1 g IV drug, 100 mg/mL concentration, ½ L IV fluid, 6 hours, IV set calibration 10 gtt/mL
J) 2 grains IV drug (use 60 mg = 1 grain), 480 mg/mL concentration, ¼ L IV fluid, 3 hours, IV set calibration 20 gtt/mL

5   Using the AAHA/AAFP guidelines for maintenance IV fluid rates for dogs (2–6 mL/kg/h) and cats (2–3 mL/kg/h), determine the minimum and maximum IV fluid flow rates in milliliters per hour for each animal:

   A) 20 kg dog
   B) 7 kg cat
   C) 43.2 kg dog
   D) 4.3 kg cat
   E) 33 lb dog
   F) 5.5 lb cat
   G) 83 lb dog
   H) 6.25 lb cat
   I) 44.25 lb dog
   J) 10.75 lb cat

6   Using the AAHA/AAFP formulas for 24 hour maintenance volume of IV fluid needed for dogs ($132 \times$ (body weight in kg)$^{0.75}$) and cats ($80 \times$ (body weight in kg)$^{0.75}$), determine what volume (in milliliters) is needed for each animal for 24 hours and what the hourly IV fluid rate (in milliliters per hour) would be needed to deliver it.

   A) 5 kg dog
   B) 5 kg cat
   C) 32.5 kg dog
   D) 3.25 kg cat
   E) 25 lb dog
   F) 8.5 lb cat
   G) 64.5 lb dog
   H) 12.1 lb cat

7   Given the estimated percentage of clinical dehydration of the patient and the weight of the animal, determine the volume of fluid needed to replace the fluid lost from dehydration in 24 hours and add that to the fluid volume needed for maintenance IV fluid for 24 hours (use 2 mL/kg/h as the maintenance IV fluid calculation for both dog and cat). List the total volume needed for maintenance and dehydration replacement combined, the rate (in mL/h and mL/min) needed to deliver the required fluid in 24 hours, and the drip per minute rate needed given the IV set calibration.

   A) 10 kg dog, 8% dehydrated, IV set calibration 15 gtt/mL
   B) 4 kg cat, 10% dehydrated, IV set calibration 60 gtt/mL
   C) 44 lb dog, 6% dehydrated, IV set calibration 20 gtt/mL
   D) 10 lb cat, 8% dehydrated, IV set calibration 20 gtt/mL
   E) 75.5 lb dog, 8% dehydrated, IV set calibration 10 gtt/mL
   F) 5.25 lb cat, 10% dehydrated, IV set calibration 60 gtt/mL
   G) 23.5 kg dog, 6% dehydrated, IV set calibration 15 gtt/mL
   H) 2.25 kg cat, 8% dehydrated, IV set calibration 20 gtt/mL

8 Given the volume of fluid to be delivered, the infusion rate, and the start time (24-hour clock times do not have an a.m. or p.m.), determine the stop time in both 12- and 24-hour clock nomenclature:

A) 450 mL, 2 mL/min infusion rate, starts at 03:10 p.m.
B) 1200 mL, 5 mL/min infusion rate, starts at 10:55 a.m.
C) 900 mL, 3 mL/min infusion rate, starts at 13:35
D) 2.2 L, 4 mL/min infusion rate, starts at 19:25
E) 1.15 L, 2.5 mL/min infusion rate, starts at 23:45
F) 0.035 L, 0.125 mL/min, 03:55

Section IV

Other Calculations Used in Veterinary Medicine

10

Ratios, Proportions, and Dilutions

OBJECTIVES
The student will be able to: 1) describe what having a ratio and a proportion means, and how these are represented mathematically, 2) use ratios mathematically to calculate unknowns, 3) define and describe the relationship between solutes, diluents/solvents, and diluted solutions, 4) describe the way dilutions and proportions may be mathematically described, 5) describe and make appropriate calculations for performing serial dilutions to achieve desired dilutions, 6) determine the volume of diluent needed to produce a specific dose or drug concentration, 7) use the $V_1 \times C_1 = V_2 \times C_2$ formula to make accurate dilutions, 8) make dilutions using concentrations described as percentage solutions, ratios, or mg/mL.

10.1   Ratios and Proportions

Ratios and proportions describe the mathematical relationship between two things:

- a ratio is a comparison between two separate items, for example milligram of drug and milliliters of liquid expressed as a concentration
- a proportion is the relationship between two ratios, for example a concentration as one ratio and the proportional milligrams of drug for a certain number of milliliters as the second ratio.

Ratios are a way of saying "x is related to y" in some manner. Ratios are expressed as fractions (like the fractions used in the conversion factors used throughout this text), or with the use of a colon as in "$x : y$" where the colon stands for the phrase "is related to."

The ratio relationships illustrated in previous chapters have been represented as a fraction with one item being the numerator and the other related item being the denominator. Because the items are equivalent to each other (e.g. 15 drips are equivalent to 1 mL for an IV set with a calibration of 15 gtt equals 1 mL) the fraction representing the ratio of "15 gtt : 1 mL" can be represented either as "15 gtt/1 mL" or as "1 mL/15 gtt." This property of ratios allows flipping ratio fractions upside down as necessary to arrange equations appropriately for use with the cancel-out method of calculations (e.g. flipping "15 gtt/mL" to "1 mL/15 gtt" if the drip units need to be canceled out).

Proportions describe the relationship between two ratios and were key to using the proportion method for performing dosage calculations. If 1 mL of a liquid is equivalent to 15 drips passing through a drip chamber

Medical Mathematics and Dosage Calculations for Veterinary Technicians, Third Edition. Robert Bill.
© 2019 John Wiley & Sons, Inc. Published 2019 by John Wiley & Sons, Inc.
Companion website: www.wiley.com/go/bill/calculations

(ratio #1), then 30 drips passing through the drip chamber must be equal to 2 mL (ratio #2). Ratio #1 is proportional to ratio #2 and therefore they can be set up as an equality:

$$\frac{15\,\text{gtt}}{1\,\text{mL}} = \frac{30\,\text{gtt}}{2\,\text{mL}}$$

The proportional method of calculating dosages uses two ratios proportional to each other, but with one component missing and represented by the unknown X unit in the proportional calculation.

$$\frac{\text{unknown}\,X\,\text{unit}}{\text{known value unit}} = \frac{\text{conversion factor with same units as unknown}\,X}{\text{conversion factor with same units as known value}}$$

For example, if an animal weighs 10 pounds and its weight needs to be converted to the equivalent kilogram body weight, two ratios are set up in a proportion. The first ratio is the "1 kg equals 2.2 lb" expressed as a fraction to represent the relationship between kilogram body weight and pound body weight. The other ratio has the missing unknown X, which is the kilogram weight of this particular animal when given the known value unit of the animal's weight in pounds (10 lb for this example). In the proportion, the units of the ratio fractions must be arranged such that the numerators on either side of the equal sign have the same units (e.g. kg) and the denominator units also are the same (e.g. lb). The unknown X always goes on the top of the equation in the proportional method, so for this example the kilograms will be the units in the numerator for both fractions.

$$\frac{\text{unknown}\,X\,\text{kg}}{10\,\text{lb}} = \frac{1\,\text{kg}}{2.2\,\text{lb}}$$

There is another way that proportional relationships between two ratios can be written. The example shown below states that the ratio of unknown X kilogram weight and a 10 pound animal is proportional to the ratio of 1 kg to 2.2 pounds.

$$\text{unknown}\,X\,\text{kg} : 10\,\text{lb} :: 1\,\text{kg} : 2.2\,\text{lb}$$

The double set of colon marks "::" indicates that the two ratios are proportional to each other. If presented with a proportion written in this format, the veterinary technician can reassemble the proportions into two ratios on either side of an equal sign to solve for unknown X (the proportion method) or use the cancel-out method by putting the unknown X by itself on the left side of the equal sign in the calculation.

$$\text{unknown}\,X\,\text{kg} : 10\,\text{lb} :: 1\,\text{kg} : 2.2\,\text{lb}$$

$$\frac{\text{unknown}\,X\,\text{kg}}{10\,\text{lb}} = \frac{1\,\text{kg}}{2.2\,\text{lb}}$$

$$\text{unknown}\,X\,\text{kg} = \frac{1\,\text{kg}}{2.2\,\text{lb}} \times 10\,\text{lb}$$

$$\text{unknown}\,X\,\text{kg} = \frac{1\,\text{kg}}{2.2\,\cancel{\text{lb}}} \times 10\,\cancel{\text{lb}}$$

$$\text{unknown}\,X\,\text{kg} = \frac{1\,\text{kg} \times 10}{2.2}$$

$$\text{unknown}\,X\,\text{kg} = 4.545\,\text{kg}$$

Thus, the ratio of 1 kg : 2.2 lb is proportionally equivalent to the ratio 4.545 kg : 10 lb. Or, as stated previously, "1 kg is to 2.2 lb as 4.545 kg is to 10 lb." This proportional property of two ratios will be used in the next section to determine equivalent solutions when doing dilutions or compounding solutions.

10.2   The Basics of Making a Dilution

Dilutions refer to a ratio of a *solute* (e.g. a drug, chemical, or other substance) mixed with a fluid or *diluent* (e.g. IV fluids) called the *solvent*. The mixture of the solute and the solvent/diluent is called the *diluted solution*. The ratio of this dilution to original solute would be represented as:

number of parts of the solute : total parts in the diluted solution

A 1 : 10 liquid dilution is also called a 1 : 10 volume-to-volume dilution because it is made up of 1 part original liquid solute (such as a liquid form of a drug) mixed with 9 parts of a liquid solvent/diluent (such as IV fluid or saline solution) to produce a total of 10 parts of diluted solution. A 1 : 10 dilution is shown graphically in Figure 10.1. A 1 : 10 dilution of the original solute means the solute will be diluted to 1/10th of its original strength. For example, if 1 mL of the original liquid solute containing 80 mg (i.e. drug concentration is 80 mg/mL) is mixed with 9 mL of a solvent/diluent such as water, 80 mg of drug is now dissolved in a larger 10 mL of the final diluted solution. The concentration of the diluted solution is 80 mg of drug in 10 mL of fluid and can be represented as the ratio fraction 80 mg/10 mL. 80 mg/10 mL reduces to 8 mg/mL, reflecting a 1/10th dilution of the original 80 mg/mL concentration.

Figure 10.1

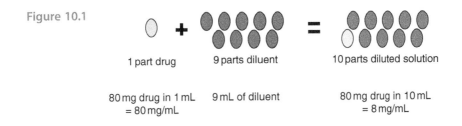

The hardest part for most students when they first begin working with dilutions is that they think of ratios such as "1 : 10" as being 1 part original solute with 10 parts of the solvent/diluent. No! The larger part of the ratio (e.g. the 10 in the 1 : 10 ratio) always refers to the *total* volume of the final diluted solution, not to the parts of the solvent diluent.

Ratios for dilution don't necessarily have to be "one to something" but can be 5 : 15, 2 : 10, 4 : 25, etc. For a 5 : 15 ratio dilution, the original solute would be 5 parts and the final diluted solution would be 15 parts. To determine the amount of solvent/diluent that must be added to the original solute to make the diluted solution, the parts of the original solute (5) would be subtracted from total number of parts of the total diluted solution (15). 15 minus 5 equals 10 parts of solvent/diluent needed. If each "part" in the previous example was 1 mL (e.g. 5 parts equals 5 mL) then the actual volume of solvent/diluent added to the original solute would have been 10 mL. Knowing the parts of the solute, the parts of the final diluted solution, and determining the parts of the solvent/diluent will be a recurring calculation used for all dilution problems.

Here is an example of how this applies to diluting a drug to give to a patient. A veterinarian wants the veterinary technician to take 1 mL of a 500 mg/mL drug solution and dilute it with enough sterile water to produce a 5 mg/mL solution for a patient. What volume of diluent/solvent would have to be added to the original solute (1 mL of 500 mg/mL) to produce a final diluted solution of 5 mg/mL? The first question to be answered is what dilution ratio has been ordered? The original concentration was 500 mg/mL and the final dilution is only 5 mg/mL which is 1/100th of the original. Therefore this must be a 1 : 100 dilution. If the ratio were not readily apparent, it could be determined by simply dividing the larger number by the smaller number (e.g. 500 divided by 5 = 100 so it is a 1 : 100 dilution). Once the 1 : 100 ratio has been determined, the volume of the final diluted solution can be determined. By definition, if the original solute was 1 part of the 1 : 100 ratio (pre-scribed as 1 mL of the 500 mg/mL drug), the final diluted solution would have to be 100 corresponding parts. Therefore, the final diluted solution volume must be 100 mL. Now that the volume of the original solute and final solution are determined, the volume of diluent/solvent is calculated by subtracting the final original solute volume from the final diluted volume.

number of total parts – number of original solute parts = number of solvent parts

100 mL total – 1 mL original solute = 99 mL solvent

Adding 99 mL of sterile water to 1 mL of the original 500 mg/mL drug would yield the final solution with the required 1 : 100 dilution containing 5 mg/mL of drug. Understanding this concept is very important before proceeding onto the next sections in which serial dilutions and creation of specific volumes or concentrations of product from stock solutions will be performed.

10.3 Making Serial Dilutions

Large dilutions are sometimes required to perform diagnostic tests or convert a concentrated drug solute into a safe and useable form. If a 1 : 10 000 dilution was required of a stock solute, 1 mL of the original stock solute would have to be mixed with 9999 mL of the diluent. However, 9999 mL is almost 10 L of liquid and it is doubtful that 10 L of the final diluted product would be needed. An alternative to performing a single large volume dilution is to perform multiple dilutions on the same solute, a process referred to as performing *serial dilutions*.

Serial dilutions are a repeated series of steps in which a solute is initially diluted with a solvent/diluent, then a small sample of the resulting diluted solution is further diluted with more solvent/diluent a second time and the process repeated until the desired dilution is obtained. For example, 1 mL of solute mixed with 9 mL of solvent/diluent yields 10 mL of a 1 : 10 diluted solution containing 1/10th the concentration of the original solute. Taking 1 mL of the diluted solution and mixing it with 9 mL of solvent/diluent would dilute the solute by another 1 : 10 ratio and yield 10 mL of a final solution that was 1/100th the concentration of the original solute. The process may be repeated until a 1 : 1000, 1 : 10 000, or 1 : 1 000 000 diluted final solution is obtained. Mathematically, this serial dilution can be represented by multiplying each dilution as a fraction, as shown below.

original solute concentration × dilutions = diluted final solution concentration

original solute concentration $\times \dfrac{1}{10} \times \dfrac{1}{10} \times \dfrac{1}{10}$ = diluted final solution concentration

If the veterinary technician was required to create a 0.5 mg/mL solution from a 500 mg/mL concentration of drug in a stock bottle, performing a serial dilution would be one way of creating the diluted final solution. Again, the first step is to determine the final dilution from the original solute. In this case 500 divided by 0.5 equals 1000 so the dilution is 1 : 1000 or 1/1000th of the original concentration. The serial dilution can be done as a series of 1 : 10 dilutions until the desired concentration is achieved.

original solute concentration × dilutions = diluted final solution concentration

$$\frac{500\,mg}{mL} \times \frac{1}{10} \times \frac{1}{10} \times \frac{1}{10} = \text{diluted final solution concentration}$$

$$\frac{500\,mg}{mL} \times \frac{1}{10} \times \frac{1}{10} \times \frac{1}{10} = \frac{500\,mg}{1000\,mL}$$

$$\frac{500\,mg}{mL} \times \frac{1}{10} \times \frac{1}{10} \times \frac{1}{10} = \frac{0.5\,mg}{mL}$$

Three serial dilutions of 1 : 10 would be needed to produce the correct final diluted solution concentration. The number of steps could be reduced if 1 : 100 dilutions were used instead of two of the 1 : 10 dilutions. A 1 : 100 dilution would be 0.1 mL of the original solution diluted by 9.9 mL of solvent/diluent to yield 10.0 mL of final solution at 1/100th of the original solution. If 1 mL of this diluted solution was then diluted additionally with 9 mL of solvent/diluent again, the final diluted solution would be 10 mL of liquid at 1/1000 the original solute concentration.

$$\frac{500\,mg}{mL} \times \frac{1}{100} \times \frac{1}{10} = \frac{500\,mg}{1000\,mL} = \frac{0.5\,mg}{mL}$$

10.4 Calculating Diluent Needed to Deliver a Specific Dose or Drug Concentration

The basic concept of determining the volume of the diluent to be added to the solute to achieve the desired final solution as described above is key to performing calculations with dilutions. This concept can be applied to calculate what volume of a concentrated solute and volume of solvent/diluent is needed to achieve a prescribed volume of a new diluted solution.

For example, the veterinary technician calculated an IV infusion cancer drug dose for a dog to be 500 mg. The drug to be infused is very irritating to the veins so the veterinarian wants to infuse the drug at a diluted concentration of 5 mg/mL. Because the cancer drug is a human drug and manufactured for human use, it does not come in a convenient 5 mg/mL concentration for animals. Instead, the concentration of the human drug concentration is 20 mg/mL. Thus, this 20 mg/mL concentration must be appropriately diluted to make a 5 mg/mL concentration.

The solution to this problem is to first determine the volume of the 20 mg/mL drug required to deliver the 500 mg dose using the techniques explained in earlier chapters for all liquid dosage forms. Then that volume of 20 mg/mL drug must be appropriately diluted to deliver it as 5 mg/mL concentration. For the first step the unknown X is the volume of liquid drug needed to deliver the dose, the known value is the dose of 500 mg, and the conversion is the concentration of the drug 20 mg/mL.

$$\text{unknown } X \text{ unit} = \text{known value unit} \times \frac{\text{conversion factor with same units as unknown } X}{\text{conversion factor with same units as known value}}$$

$$X \text{ mL volume needed} = 500\,mg\,dose \times \frac{1\,mL}{20\,mg}$$

$$X \text{ mL volume needed} = 500\,\cancel{mg} \times \frac{1\,mL}{20\,\cancel{mg}}$$

$$X \text{ mL volume needed} = \frac{500 \times 1\,\text{mL}}{20}$$

$$X \text{ mL volume needed} = \frac{500\,\text{mL}}{20}$$

$$X \text{ mL volume needed} = 25\,\text{mL}$$

Now that is it known that 25 mL of the 20 mg/mL concentration is needed to deliver 500 mg dose of the drug, the 25 mL must be diluted to produce a 5 mg/mL concentration. The ratio of dilution from 20 mg/mL to 5 mg/mL is first determined by dividing 20 by 5 to give 4. Thus, the dilution required to go from 20 mg/mL to 5 mg/mL is a 1 : 4 dilution. The original volume of solute parts (volume of the original concentrated solution) is 25 mL, which means that the number of total parts of the final 1 : 4 diluted solution must be four times 25 mL which equals 100 mL. Having determined the total milliliters needed for the final diluted solution (100 mL equals total parts) and having calculated the volume of the original solute needed (25 mL), the volume of solvent needed to dilute the drug is the difference between the total (100 mL) and the volume accounted for by the original solution (25 mL).

number of total parts – number of original solute parts = number of solvent parts

volume of total parts – volume of original solution parts = volume of diluent

100 mL – 25 mL = volume of diluent

100 mL – 25 mL = 75 mL

The 25 mL of the 20 mg/mL solution needed to deliver the 500 mg of drug needs to be diluted with 75 mL of solvent/diluent (such as sterile water or isotonic saline) to produce 100 mL of 5 mg/mL solution.

10.5 Calculating Dilutions Using the $V_1 \times C_1 = V_2 \times C_2$ Formula

Veterinary technicians often are asked to create diluted volumes of disinfectants, IV solutions, or medication from more concentrated "stock" bottles. For example, if the original stock solution of a drug is 400 mg/mL and the veterinarian wants the patient to receive 250 mL of a diluted 20 mg/mL solution of the drug, how much IV fluid solvent/diluent has to be added to what volume of the more concentrated 400 mg/mL drug to produce 250 mL of the diluted solution? The answer to this can be determined using the milligram dose of drug needed and the process that was described previously. However, there is another calculation that is commonly found in medical math and chemistry books that can be used to determine how to create the diluted solution. The equation is: $V_1 \times C_1 = V_2 \times C_2$

V_1 = volume of the more concentrated solution (original solute)
V_2 = volume of the more diluted solution (final diluted solution)
C_1 = concentration of the more concentrated solution (original solute concentration)
C_2 = concentration of the more diluted solution (final diluted solution concentration)

In the example problem, the volume of the final diluted solution (V_2) is 250 mL and the concentration of the diluted solution is 20 mg/mL (C_2). The original, more concentrated stock solution is 400 mg/mL (C_1), but the volume of the stock solution needed to the create the dilution is yet unknown (V_1). This V_1 can be determined using the $V_1 \times C_1 = V_2 \times C_2$ equation, and then the V_1 and V_2 together can be used to determine the amount of diluent that needs to be added to the original concentrated solute.

$$V_1 \times C_1 = V_2 \times C_2$$

$$V_1 \times \frac{400\,\text{mg}}{\text{mL}} = 250\,\text{mL} \times \frac{20\,\text{mg}}{\text{mL}}$$

The equation is rearranged mathematically to leave V_1 on the left side of the equation by itself by multiplying both sides of the equation by the reciprocal of 400 mg/mL.

$$V_1 \times \frac{400\,\text{mg}}{\text{mL}} \times \frac{\text{mL}}{400\,\text{mg}} = 250\,\text{mL} \times \frac{20\,\text{mg}}{\text{mL}} \times \frac{\text{mL}}{400\,\text{mg}}$$

$$V_1 \times \frac{400\,\cancel{\text{mg}}}{\cancel{\text{mL}}} \times \frac{\cancel{\text{mL}}}{400\,\cancel{\text{mg}}} = 250\,\text{mL} \times \frac{20\,\cancel{\text{mg}}}{\cancel{\text{mL}}} \times \frac{\cancel{\text{mL}}}{400\,\cancel{\text{mg}}}$$

$$V_1 \times \frac{400}{400} = 250\,\text{mL} \times \frac{20}{400}$$

$$V_1 \times 1 = 250\,\text{mL} \times 0.05$$

$$V_1 = 12.5\,\text{mL}$$

12.5 mL of the original concentrated 400 mg/mL drug solution (the solute) is needed for the final 250 mL solution. The remainder of the 250 mL diluted solution is made up of diluent (for example IV fluids, sterile saline, sterile water). 250 mL minus 12.5 mL of original concentrated drug leaves 237.5 mL to be made up by the diluent.

The formula can be used to determine any of the other variables V_2, C_1, or C_2 if three of the four variables are known. For example, if the veterinary technician knows the volume and concentration of the original concentrated stock solution (variables V_1 and C_1), and knows how much diluent is going to be added to the stock solution, then V_2 (the volume of the final diluted solution) can be determined ($V_2 = V_1 +$ diluent volume). Once V_1, C_1, and V_2 are known, the concentration of the final diluted solution (C_2) can be calculated using the formula.

For example, 25 mL of a 10 mg/mL stock reagent solution (the original solution) is going to be added to 100 mL of a diluent. What will be the concentration of the final diluted solution (C_2)? V_1 is provided (25 mL) as is C_1 (10 mg/mL). The final volume V_2 is calculated by adding the V_1 to the amount of diluent (100 mL); V_2 equals 25 mL plus 100 mL for a total of 125 mL. Three of the four variables are now defined (V_1, C_1, V_2) so the last variable, the concentration of the final solution (C_2), can be calculated.

$$V_1 \times C_1 = V_2 \times C_2$$

$$25\,\text{mL} \times \frac{200\,\text{mg}}{\text{mL}} = 125\,\text{mL} \times \frac{???\,\text{mg}}{\text{mL}}$$

The variable to be solved is isolated on one side of the equation by mathematically "moving" everything else to the other side of the equation using reciprocal multiplication.

$$25\,\text{mL} \times \frac{200\,\text{mg}}{\text{mL}} \times \frac{1}{125\,\text{mL}} = 125\,\text{mL} \times \frac{1}{125\,\text{mL}} \times \frac{???\text{mg}}{\text{mL}}$$

$$25\,\cancel{\text{mL}} \times \frac{200\,\text{mg}}{\text{mL}} \times \frac{1}{125\,\cancel{\text{mL}}} = 125\,\cancel{\text{mL}} \times \frac{1}{125\,\cancel{\text{mL}}} \times \frac{???\text{mg}}{\text{mL}}$$

$$\frac{200\,\text{mg}}{\text{mL}} \times \frac{25}{125} = \frac{125}{125} \times \frac{???\text{mg}}{\text{mL}}$$

$$\frac{200\,\text{mg}}{\text{mL}} \times 0.2 = 1 \times \frac{???\text{mg}}{\text{mL}}$$

$$\frac{40\,\text{mg}}{\text{mL}} = \frac{???\text{mg}}{\text{mL}}$$

The final solution concentration will be 40 mg/mL.

To summarize, the $V_1 \times C_1 = V_2 \times C_2$ equation can be used to determine any of the variables as long as the other three variables are known. To work this equation, the amount of diluent that is to be added to the original concentrated solution must either be given to determine V_2 (V_2 equals V_1 plus volume of diluent), or the equation is used to determine amount of diluent that needs to be added by having or calculating both V_2 and V_1 (volume of diluent equals V_2 minus V_1). This relationship between V_1, V_2, and the volume of diluent is the same concept emphasized at the beginning of this chapter:

number of total parts = number of original solute parts + number of solvent parts

volume of final solution = volume original solute + volume of solvent or diluent

10.6 Diluting Percent Solutions

Many disinfectants and some medications are not listed by milligram per milliliter, but by their percent solution (e.g. 3% solution). The definition and conversion of percent solutions to mg/mL concentrations were explained in Chapter 7. The calculation of percent solution dilutions uses the same concepts as described above, but may require an additional step of converting the percent solution to milligrams per milliliter.

A veterinarian wants to dilute a more concentrated 5% antiseptic solution to 250 mL of a milder 2% solution. How much of the original 5% solution is needed, and what is the volume of diluent needed to produce 250 mL of the more dilute solution? The definition of a percent solution is "X grams of solute per 100 mL of solvent," or put another way, X grams of drug/active ingredient dissolved in 100 mL of some liquid. Thus, a 5% solution would be 5 g (*not* milligrams) of active ingredient of the antiseptic dissolved in 100 mL (*not* 1 mL) of liquid, and the 2% solution would be 2 g per 100 mL of liquid. As described in Chapter 7, the grams per 100 mL were converted to milligrams per milliliter (mg/mL) either by conversion math (grams to milligrams) or by the short cut of adding a zero to the original percent numeral. Thus, 5% is equivalent to 50 mg/mL and 2% is equivalent to 20 mg/mL. Once these percent solutions are in the "mg/mL" format, the $V_1 \times C_1 = V_2 \times C_2$

formula can be used as previously described. V_1 is the unknown volume of the original concentrated 5% solution, but the other three variables (C_1, V_2, C_2) have been stated.

$$V_1 \times C_1 = V_2 \times C_2$$

$$???\text{mL} \times \frac{50\,\text{mg}}{\text{mL}} = 250\,\text{mL} \times \frac{20\,\text{mg}}{\text{mL}}$$

$$???\text{mL} \times \frac{50\,\text{mg}}{\text{mL}} \times \frac{\text{mL}}{50\,\text{mg}} = 250\,\text{mL} \times \frac{20\,\text{mg}}{\text{mL}} \times \frac{\text{mL}}{50\,\text{mg}}$$

$$???\text{mL} = 250\,\text{mL} \times \frac{20}{50}$$

$$???\text{mL} = 100\,\text{mL}$$

100 mL of the original, concentrated solution is needed. The amount of diluent to be added to the concentrated solution to achieve a total of 250 mL for the final diluted solution will be 150 mL (250–100 = 150). Thus, 100 mL of the 5% solution plus 150 mL of a diluent will produce the 250 mL of a 2% solution, as requested.

It is also possible to perform the $V_1 \times C_1 = V_2 \times C_2$ calculation using the actual percent numerals (5 and 2) for the concentrations C_1 and C_2 instead of doing the conversion from percent solution to mg/mL.

$$V_1 \times C_1 = V_2 \times C_2$$

$$???\text{mL} \times 5 = 250\,\text{mL} \times 2$$

$$???\text{mL} \times 5 \times \frac{1}{5} = 250\,\text{mL} \times 2 \times \frac{1}{5}$$

$$???\text{mL} = 250\,\text{mL} \times \frac{2}{5}$$

$$???\text{mL} = 100\,\text{mL}$$

10.7 Diluting Solutions Expressed as Ratios

If a disinfectant is a 2 : 25 solution and a veterinarian wants the veterinary technician to create 500 mL of a 1 : 40 diluted solution from it, how would this be calculated? The key is remembering that 2 : 25 is a ratio and that can be expressed as a fraction 2/25. The "2/25" concentration (C_1) doesn't have to have any units (e.g. mg or mL) attached to it as long as the diluted concentration C_2 likewise does not have units attached to it. So, 1 : 40 can be represented by the fraction 1/40 and can be used in the $V_1 \times C_1 = V_2 \times C_2$ equation in this form. In this problem C_1, V_2, and C_2 are all identified and V_1 (volume of the original concentration) and the amount of diluent to be added are unknown.

$$V_1 \times C_1 = V_2 \times C_2$$

$$??? \text{mL} \times \frac{2}{25} = 500 \text{ mL} \times \frac{1}{40}$$

$$??? \text{mL} \times \frac{2}{25} \times \frac{25}{2} = 500 \text{ mL} \times \frac{1}{40} \times \frac{25}{2}$$

$$??? \text{mL} = 500 \text{ mL} \times \frac{25}{40 \times 2}$$

$$??? \text{mL} = 500 \text{ mL} \times 0.3125$$

$$??? \text{mL} = 156.25 \text{ mL}$$

V_1 is 156.25 mL of the original 2 : 25 concentrated disinfectant to which 343.75 mL of water is added to produce 500 mL of 1 : 40 diluted final solution.

10.8 Making Dilutions with Mixed Types of Concentrations

What if the original stock solution of disinfectant is listed as a 1 : 25 dilution and the protocol calls for a diluted 2% solution of disinfectant to be used? Or what if the concentration of drug is listed as a 12.5% solution and the veterinarian wants to infuse a diluted concentration of 25 mg/mL intravenously? These problems can all be solved in the same way as the previous examples, but only after both the original solute concentration and the diluted solution concentrations are made into congruent formats (e.g. either both expressed as % solution or both expressed as mg/mL).

A ratio (e.g. 1 : 25) can be converted into a percent by knowing that 1 : 25 is equivalent to the fraction 1/25, and, as explained in Chapter 1, fractions can be converted to decimals and then into percentages by dividing the numerator by the denominator (i.e. dividing 1 by 25 in the fraction 1/25).

$$1 : 25 = \frac{1}{25}$$

$$\frac{1}{25} = 1 \div 25 = 0.04$$

$$0.04 = 4\%$$

Furthermore, a 4% solution can be converted into mg/mL by the definition of percent solution:

$$X\% \text{solution} = \frac{X \text{ grams}}{100 \text{ mL}}$$

$$4\% \text{solution} = \frac{4 \text{ grams}}{100 \text{ mL}}$$

$$\frac{4 \text{ grams}}{100 \text{ mL}} = \frac{4000 \text{ mg}}{100 \text{ mL}} = \frac{40 \text{ mg}}{\text{mL}}$$

By converting one or both concentrations into similar formats, the $V_1 \times C_1 = V_2 \times C_2$ equation can still be used to determine what volumes or concentrations are needed to make appropriate dilutions.

10.9 Chapter 10 Practice Problems

1 For each proportion, solve for the unknown X:

A) $2 : 5 :: X : 25$
B) $10 : 24 :: 15 : X$
C) $2.5 \, mg : 1 \, mL :: X \, mg : 12 \, mL$
D) $X \, mg : 12 \, mL :: 64 \, mg : 6 \, mL$
E) $7.5 \, mg : X \, mL :: 17.25 \, mg : 18.4 \, mL$

2 For each dilution, describe how many parts are solute, diluent/solvent, and final solution:

A) $1 : 20$
B) $1 : 320$
C) $2 : 5$
D) $5 : 40$
E) $10 : 250$

3 Given the original solution concentration and the serial dilutions performed on the original concentration, calculate the final solution concentration, listing the answer in milligrams per milliliter (mg/mL):

A) $200 \, mg/mL$, diluted $1 : 10, 1 : 10, 1 : 10$
B) 4% solution, diluted $1 : 20, 1 : 10$
C) $10 \, g/L$, diluted $1 : 5, 1 : 10$
D) 7.5% solution, diluted $5 : 20, 1 : 10$
E) $0.5 \, mg/mL$, diluted $4 : 25, 2 : 3, 1 : 10$

4 Given the volume and concentration of the original concentrated solution and the dilution required for the diluted final solution, state the volume and concentration of the final diluted solution and the amount of diluent used to produce the correct dilution:

A) $15 \, mL$ of $50 \, mg/mL$ needs a $1 : 4$ dilution
B) $2.5 \, mL$ of $100 \, mg/mL$ needs a $2 : 10$ dilution
C) $50 \, mL$ of $25 \, mg/mL$ needs a $2 : 5$ dilution
D) $3.5 \, mL$ of $12.5 \, mg/mL$ needs a $3 : 12$ dilution
E) $4 \, mL$ of 3% solution needs a $5 : 8$ dilution

5 Using the $V_1 \times C_1 = V_2 \times C_2$ equation, determine the volume of original solution and the amount of diluent needed to produce the prescribed volume of the final diluted solution:

A) $100 \, mg/mL$ original solution concentration, need $125 \, mL$ of $25 \, mg/mL$ final diluted solution
B) $50 \, mg/mL$ original solution concentration, need $40 \, mL$ of $10 \, mg/mL$ final diluted solution
C) $240 \, mg/mL$ original solution concentration, need $100 \, mL$ of $60 \, mg/mL$ final diluted solution
D) $0.5 \, mg/mL$ original solution concentration, need $4 \, mL$ of $0.025 \, mg/mL$ final diluted solution
E) 8% original solution concentration, need $250 \, mL$ of 4% solution for final diluted solution
F) 50% original solution concentration, need $500 \, mL$ of 15% solution for final diluted solution
G) 37.5% original solution concentration, need $100 \, mL$ of 6% solution for final diluted solution
H) 4% original solution concentration, need $25 \, mL$ of 0.5% solution for final diluted solution
I) 25.0% original solution concentration, need $250 \, mL$ of 0.125% solution for final diluted solution
J) $1 : 2$ original solution concentration, need $100 \, mL$ of $1 : 4$ final diluted solution

    K) 1 : 5 original solution concentration, need 200 mL of 1 : 8 final diluted solution

    L) 4 : 5 original solution concentration, need 250 mL of 1 : 2 final diluted solution

    M) 2 : 3 original solution concentration, need 120 mL of 1 : 3 final diluted solution

6   Using the $V_1 \times C_1 = V_2 \times C_2$ equation, solve each of the problems:

    A) If 2 mL of 100 mg/mL is added to 20 mL of diluent, what is the volume and concentration of the final diluted solution?

    B) What volume of the stock disinfectant with a concentration of 30 mg/mL and volume of diluent must be added together to produce 200 mL of a 15 mg/mL final diluted solution?

    C) A technician is reading a recipe for creating 240 mL of a 2% diluted reagent. She can tell that 80 mL of diluent is used to make the final diluted reagent solution, but can't read the volume or concentration of the original concentrated reagent solution needed. What is the volume and concentration of the original reagent (in % solution and in mg/mL) needed?

    D) 10 mL of a 320 mg/mL concentrated solution needs to be diluted to a 20 mg/mL solution. What volume of diluent is needed and what is the volume of the final diluted solution?

7   Using the $V_1 \times C_1 = V_2 \times C_2$ equation, solve each of the problems:

    A) What volume of concentrated 24% solution and volume of diluent is needed to make 150 mL of 1 : 10 diluted solution?

    B) 12 mL of a 640 mg/mL concentration of drug needs to be diluted to 1 : 2 solution. What is the volume of diluent and volume of final diluted solution?

    C) What volume and concentration of drug (in mg/mL) is needed to be mixed with 100 mL of diluent to produce 400 mL of a diluted 6% solution?

    D) A 480 mg/mL concentrated drug form needs to be diluted to form 300 mL of a 2% diluted solution. What volume of original drug and what volume of diluent are needed to produce the final diluted solution?

    E) 12 mL of a concentrated 5 : 8 ratio of antiseptic is diluted with 363 mL of diluent to produce what volume and percentage concentration of the final diluted solution?

11

Additional Calculations Used by Veterinary Professionals

OBJECTIVES

The student will be able to:

1) identify the mean, median, mode, and range for a data set,
2) accurately convert between the Fahrenheit and Celsius temperature scales, and
3) read and write Roman numerals.

11.1 Mean, Median, Mode, and Range

Contemporary literature in veterinary nursing or veterinary technology often contains some statistical analysis describing aspects of a scientific study. Also, information on new drugs or products will use basic statistics to "show" how one drug or product is superior to another. Thus, it is important for the veterinary technician to understand some of the common language and meanings of basic statistical results to better understand current literature and more objectively evaluate product information.

Four statistical terms commonly used, discussed, or manipulated to promote a product are the mean, median, mode, and range.

The *mean* is also the "the mathematical average." For a given set of numbers (e.g. the numerical results from multiple experiments) the mean would be determined by taking all the individual values (the individual experimental test results), adding them together, and then dividing that total by the number of tests performed. For example, a drug was being tested for how well it reduced the heart rate in dogs with a particular type of cardiac disease. The data from a small study of nine dogs is shown below, where the percent listed is the percent decrease in heart rate due to the drug (ranked in order from least effect to most effect):

Dog 1 = 7%
Dog 2 = 10%
Dog 3 = 12%
Dog 4 = 16%
Dog 5 = 17%
Dog 6 = 18%
Dog 7 = 20%
Dog 8 = 20%
Dog 9 = 24%

Medical Mathematics and Dosage Calculations for Veterinary Technicians, Third Edition. Robert Bill.
© 2019 John Wiley & Sons, Inc. Published 2019 by John Wiley & Sons, Inc.
Companion website: www.wiley.com/go/bill/calculations

The mean decreased heart rate for these nine dogs was determined by adding all the individual percent numbers together and dividing by the total number of dogs.

$$\frac{(7 + 10 + 12 + 16 + 17 + 18 + 20 + 20 + 24)}{9 \, \text{dogs}} = 16 \, \text{mean}$$

For this population of nine dogs, the drug decreased the heart rate by a mean of 16%.

The *median* is the middle number in the range of numbers when they are arranged from lowest to highest value. In this example of nine dogs, there are 9 numbers arranged in order in the list and the middle number of the set would be the value in the #5 position, which is 17%. So the mean (average) of the drug effect for these 9 dogs is a 16% decrease and the median of the results is a 17% decrease.

To spare the need to physically count the number of results to find the middle result for the median value, a simple formula is used to determine which value, when the data is arranged from smallest to largest, will be the median. The formula is:

$$\text{median} = \frac{\text{number of data points} + 1}{2}$$

meaning that the number of data points (not their values) is added to 1 and then that sum is divided by 2. For this example, there were 9 dogs (9 data points) arranged in order from low to high so the formula is (9 + 1)/2 equals 5. Dog #5's value is the median value of the data set.

If there is an even number of data points (e.g. 10 dogs were used instead of 9 dogs), then there is no middle data point because there are 5 data points in the top half of the data set and 5 data points in the bottom half of the data set. In the situation with 10 dogs, the formula used above to determine the median data point would be: (10 + 1)/2 equals 5.5. There is no "Dog #5.5" for a data point, so the median would be the average of the two data points that flank either side of the mythical middle data point 5.5. In another example data set of numbers, below, there are 12 numbers and the median is the average of data points #6 and #7:

32	35	38	39	40	41	42	44	45	47	49	51

The median position is position 6.5, as (12 + 1)/2 equals 6.5, so the median value would be the average of data point #6 (has a value of 41) and data point #7 (has a value of 42), which means the median value is 41.5.

Shifting back to the mean, it would be nice statistically if half of the values in the data set were above the mean value and half below it, but in real data sets this rarely happens. Thus, the curve of data points rarely looks like the stereotypical "bell-shaped curve" shown in Figure 11.1. However, by looking at the median and the mean, it is possible to roughly see how the distribution of data points might be skewed towards one side of the mean or the other. In the example above with the nine dogs, the mean

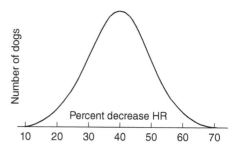

Figure 11.1 A bell-shaped curve showing number of dogs exhibiting each percent decrease in heart rate

(average) for the population of nine dogs was 16% which is less than the median value of 17%. So even though 17% represents the value of the middle data point of the sample, the average of 16% suggests that there are numerically more values pulling the mean down below the 17% median point than there are numerical values pulling the mean above 17%. Hence the data is skewed towards the lower half of the test values. In the nine-dog data set, the lowest value of the data set (7%) was much farther removed from the median (17%) than the highest value of the data set (24%) which pulls the mean (average) of the entire data set towards a point below the median point. The opposite would happen, and the mean would be above the median, if the collective deviation from the median value of the top half of data points was greater than the deviation of the bottom half data points. Looking at both the mean and the median can give an idea of how the overall population of data points may be skewed.

The *mode* means the value in the data set that is most frequently represented. If the drug study measuring the decreased heart rate in dogs used a much larger number of dogs, the results of the study would be plotted with the number of dogs on the vertical y axis of the chart and the percent decrease in heart rate plotted along the horizontal x axis. The resulting plotted curve for the number of dogs with each percent decrease in heart rate might look something like Figure 11.1.

The mode for this larger data set would be the percent decrease in heart rate that appeared in the most dogs. Looking at the bell-shaped curve shown in Figure 11.1, it appears that the mode for this study was likely the 40% decrease in heart rate because that percent is the highest point of the bell-shaped curve and represents the largest number of dogs with that percent decrease in heart rate.

Like the mean and the median, the mode of the data can also convey information about how the curve may be skewed from the ideal bell-shaped curve shown in Figure 11.1. An example for how the mode can add to the interpretation of data can be shown by contrasting two different studies on cats being tested with a drug that decreases arterial blood pressure. The first study was performed in 15 cats given a drug and the change in arterial blood pressure, expressed as percent decrease, was recorded. The data is shown below, arranged from smallest to largest percentage drop.

Cat 1 = 10%
Cat 2 = 11%
Cat 3 = 12%
Cat 4 = 13%
Cat 5 = 14%
Cat 6 = 15%
Cat 7 = 17%
Cat 8 = 19%
Cat 9 = 20%
Cat 10 = 20%
Cat 11 = 22%
Cat 12 = 24%
Cat 13 = 26%
Cat 14 = 27%
Cat 15 = 29%

The mean drop of blood pressure in this trial of 15 cats was 18.6%. (Remember that the mean equals the total of all values divided by the number of tests.) The median value for the ranked results should be the eighth value because $(15 + 1)/2 = 8$. The value for Cat #8 is 19%. Because the value of 20% is found in two cats (Cats

#9 and #10) the mode in this small study would be 20%. The mode in this small study is still located towards the middle of the data set values, which is consistent with what was shown in Figure 11.1 with a study containing many more data points.

Another blood pressure trial on 15 other cats was then performed and the data collected as before. The results for this data set are shown below. The data in the second study has the exact same mean (18.6% average drop in arterial blood pressure for the population of tested cats) and the median value of 19% is also the same as the previous set of cats.

Cat 1 = 13%
Cat 2 = 14%
Cat 3 = 15%
Cat 4 = 15%
Cat 5 = 15%
Cat 6 = 15%
Cat 7 = 16%
Cat 8 = 19%
Cat 9 = 20%
Cat 10 = 22%
Cat 11 = 22%
Cat 12 = 22%
Cat 13 = 22%
Cat 14 = 24%
Cat 15 = 25%

However, despite both trials having the same mean and median, the mode in the second trial would be very different than the mode in the first trial. In the second trial there were two sets of numbers that occurred four times, 15% and 22%, suggesting two modes or a *bimodal* distribution of the data points. The two modes were not in the middle of the data set, but towards the ends of the data set. If plotted out like in Figure 11.1 there would appear to be two humps on the curve located over 15% and 22%. The results in the second study suggest that perhaps there is another factor that affects the population of cats in this study such that one group responds above the median value and one group responds below the median value. The variation in population response between the two cat studies would not have been noticed by looking at just the mean and the median from each study, but required use of the mode or plotting out the entire data set into a curve like in Figure 11.1.

The *range* is the distance between the lowest value and the highest value in a data set. In the two small cat studies just discussed, the range for the first study was 10–29% and the range in the second study was 13–25%. Thus the range in the first study was 19 and the range in the second study was smaller or narrower at 12. The mean and median were identical between the two studies, but the first study suggests a more variable response to the drug because the range was wider than the second study. Generally, the narrower the range, the more statistically significant the results in demonstrating a particular outcome. A wider range often indicates more variable responses in the population tested and dilutes the support that the tested variable itself was alone responsible for the observed changes.

Knowing the definition and uses of the statistical terms of mean, median, mode, and range can help the veterinary technician better evaluate data being presented. Further information on important statistical terminology like *p*-value, significance, correlation, *R*-value, and standard deviation can be found in online resources or any standard introductory statistics textbook. Understanding these additional terms can further help you understand the meaning of statistical data.

11.2 Converting between Fahrenheit and Celsius

Body temperatures of veterinary patients in Canada and Europe are written as *degrees Celsius* (also sometimes still called by the older term, *degrees centigrade*), while the *Fahrenheit scale* of temperature is used in the United States, albeit less so than in the past. Digital thermometers allow easy switching between each scale when taking a patient's temperature, but the general public in the United States still refers to weather temperatures, cooking temperatures, and other common uses of temperature as degrees Fahrenheit. Because the use of both scales can be found in veterinary literature and communications with the general public, the veterinary professional should become familiar with how to accurately convert from the Fahrenheit to the Celsius (centigrade) scale, and vice versa.

The Fahrenheit scale uses 32 °F as the point at which water freezes and 212 °F as the temperature at which water boils. The Celsius scale has taken these two end points and made them 0 °C for water freezing and 100 °C for water boiling. The "centigrade" in the "degrees centigrade" scale, which is the same scale as that invented by Celsius, refers to the "100 marks" between water freezing and boiling on the centigrade scale.

Anyone who uses the Fahrenheit to Celsius conversion formula often struggles to remember how the formula is set up. However, briefly examining the mathematical proportions used by the formulas for converting between these scales will help the veterinary technician to better remember how to apply the formulas. First, notice the difference between 32 and 212 °F is 180° on the Fahrenheit scale whereas the difference between these same freezing and boiling points on the Celsius scale is only 100° (100−0 °C). If a ratio of number of Celsius increments between freezing and boiling of water and the corresponding Fahrenheit increments is made, it results in a ratio that can be converted into a fraction:

100 increments on Celsius scale : 180 increments on Fahrenheit scale

$$\frac{100\ \text{increments on Celsius scale}}{180\ \text{increments on Fahrenheit scale}}$$

$$\frac{100}{180}$$

$$\frac{5}{9}$$

The 5/9 fraction plays a key role in the formula used to convert Fahrenheit to Celsius. The reciprocal, 9/5, is used in the formula to convert Celsius to Fahrenheit. In using the formula for Fahrenheit to Celsius, the 5/9 fraction will be multiplied by a number and the result will be a smaller value because 5/9 is a fraction less than 1. When a Fahrenheit temperature value is converted to a Celsius value, the temperatures are going from a larger scale (Fahrenheit with 180 increments) to a smaller scale (Celsius with only 100 increments) and the Celsius number will always be smaller.

The 9/5 fraction would be used in the formula to convert a temperature value from Celsius to Fahrenheit because the Celsius scale expands from 100 to 180 on the Fahrenheit scale, producing a larger number after the conversion. In the Celsius to Fahrenheit conversion formula, 9/5 is used because any number multiplied by the fraction 9/5 will become larger since 9/5 is a fraction greater than 1.

The other key factor incorporated into the temperature conversion formulas is the temperatures on both scales at which water freezes. The freezing point (32 °F and 0 °C) is used as the common "baseline" of both scales, therefore, it is necessary to mathematically orient both temperature scales to this common baseline value before or after expanding or contracting the scales with 5/9 or 9/5. In converting a temperature value from Fahrenheit to Celsius, 32 must be *subtracted* from any Fahrenheit value to orient the Fahrenheit scale down to the 0 °C freezing point of the Celsius scale. Conversely, when converting from the Celsius scale to Fahrenheit, 32 must be *added* back to the Celsius temperature value to "normalize" the conversion to the freezing water temperature baseline of the Fahrenheit scale.

Thus, the conversion between the two temperature scales has two components: multiplying by the fraction 5/9 or 9/5, and adding or subtracting 32. By remembering when to use which fraction and when to subtract or add 32 points, the correct formula for converting between the two scales will make more sense and be more readily remembered.

$$\text{Celsius temperature} = (F - 32) \times \frac{5}{9}$$

$$\text{Fahrenheit temperature} = \left(C \times \frac{9}{5} \right) + 32$$

For specifically converting Fahrenheit to the equivalent Celsius temperature, 32 must first be subtracted from the Fahrenheit value to "normalize" the Fahrenheit scale to the same frozen-water baseline as the Celsius scale. Then the number must be condensed from the larger Fahrenheit scale value to the smaller Celsius scale by multiplying the normalized temperature value by 5/9.

Here is an example: if a patient's temperature is 102 °F, what is the equivalent °C?

$$\text{Celsius temperature} = (F - 32) \times \frac{5}{9}$$

$$\text{Celsius temperature} = (102 - 32) \times \frac{5}{9}$$

$$\text{Celsius temperature} = (70) \times \frac{5}{9}$$

$$\text{Celsius temperature} = \frac{70 \times 5}{9}$$

$$\text{Celsius temperature} = 38.9$$

A patient with 102 °F body temperature has a temperature of 38.9 °C.

To convert from the more compact Celsius scale to the more expansive Fahrenheit scale, first expand the Celsius value by multiplying it by the larger fraction, 9/5. Then the product of this multiplication must be reset to the baseline water freezing point for the Fahrenheit scale by adding 32 to the product of the 9/5 multiplication. Notice how the order of multiplying by the fraction and then using 32 to normalize the baseline is reversed compared with the Fahrenheit to Celsius conversion (where the 32 baseline resetting was performed first and the multiplication to condense the scale performed second).

Here is another example: what is the temperature of a water bath in Fahrenheit if the water bath temperature reads 32.5 °C?

$$\text{Fahrenheit temperature} = \left(C \times \frac{9}{5} \right) + 32$$

$$\text{Fahrenheit temperature} = \left(32.5 \times \frac{9}{5}\right) + 32$$

$$\text{Fahrenheit temperature} = \left(\frac{32.5 \times 9}{5}\right) + 32$$

$$\text{Fahrenheit temperature} = (58.5) + 32$$

$$\text{Fahrenheit temperature} = 90.5$$

Now that the temperature conversion process has been explained with these two formulas, there is a "simpler" formula that can be used mathematically so that only one formula needs be remembered for making temperature conversions both ways. That formula is shown below:

$$5F = 9C + 160$$

The F stands for the temperature in degrees Fahrenheit, the C stands for the temperature in degrees Celsius, the 160 represents the product of 5×32. The 5/9 or 9/5 fraction is represented mathematically in the new equation by being attached to the F and C variables. If there is any doubt about the validity of this "simpler" formula, both of the original conversion equations can be mathematically converted into this one equation by algebraically manipulating the components of the equations to put $5F$ by itself on one side of the equation.

Fortunately, a mnemonic device (a memory prompt) can be used to help remember part of this formula. There are "five fingers on one hand", so "$5F$" is found in the equation, and "cats have nine lives", so the nine is attached to the C as "$9C$." While this formula is easier to remember, the disadvantage of this equation is that the algebra used to solve the problem is a little more difficult. Thus, some prefer to remember the two original equations above and others prefer to use the single, simpler equation provided they have a solid grasp of how to move variables within an equation using algebra.

Examples of how to use the single equation is shown below, using the values from the examples above.

Example 1: if the patient's temperature is $102\,°F$, what is the equivalent temperature in $°C$?

$$5F = 9C + 160$$

$$5 \times 102 = 9C + 160$$

$$510 = 9C + 160$$

$$510 - 160 = 9C + 160 - 160$$

$$350 = 9C$$

$$350 \times \frac{1}{9} = 9C \times \frac{1}{9}$$

$$\frac{350}{9} = C$$

$$38.9 = C$$

Example 2: what is the temperature of the water bath in Fahrenheit if the water bath temperature reads 32.5 °C?

$$5F = 9C + 160$$

$$5F = (9 \times 32.5) + 160$$

$$5F = (292.5) + 160$$

$$5F = 452.5$$

$$5F \times \frac{1}{5} = 452.5 \times \frac{1}{5}$$

$$F \times \frac{5}{5} = \frac{452.5}{5}$$

$$F \times 1 = 90.5$$

$$F = 90.5$$

Regardless of which formulas are used, it is important to practice making these conversions to ensure that the calculations are performed correctly 100% of the time. A good way to practice this is to take the normal temperature ranges of common domestic animals and convert them to the scale that is less familiar. If Fahrenheit is more familiar, convert the temperatures into Celsius, or vice versa. Once converted, memorize the common body temperatures in both scales so that body temperatures in both scales are immediately recognized as normal or abnormal.

Table 11.1 shows Fahrenheit and Celsius values for a range of temperatures.

Table 11.1 Samples of commonly used temperatures in Fahrenheit and Celsius

Fahrenheit	Celsius
0	−17.8
32	0.0
50	10.0
90	32.2
98.6	37
100	37.8
101	38.3
102	38.9
103	39.4
104	40.0
212	100

11.3 Roman Numerals

Occasionally, Roman numeral nomenclature appears in everyday life or medical literature. For example, many movies, television shows, and videos list their copyright date at the end of the film in Roman numerals. Examples are MCMXCVII (which is 1997) or MMXVIII (which is 2018). Major sporting events such as the Olympics and the Super Bowl designate themselves using Roman numerals, so that Olympics XXIII is the 23rd Olympics and Super Bowl LII is Super Bowl 52. Volumes of journals or scientific literature may be indexed according to Roman numerals as in "Vol XIV, number 2"; or the page numbers of the opening portion of a textbook may be represented as lower case Roman numerals (e.g. viii is page 8).

Perhaps the most commonly encountered Roman numerals in veterinary medicine are the numerals found on the front of the boxes of controlled substance or Schedule drugs, where the Roman numerals are used to indicate the abuse potential of the drug. Schedule drugs are required by law to have a large "C" and a Roman numeral clearly displayed on the drug label to indicate the abuse potential and to signal to the veterinarian and veterinary technician the special storage requirements or tracking of the drug's use in the hospital. The controlled substance designations run from C-II (most abuse potential for drugs that can be legally prescribed) to C-V (pronounced "see-five"), which are drugs with the least abuse potential. C-I drugs are those drugs with abuse potentials so high that they are considered to have "no legitimate medicinal value." Such C-I drugs would include LSD, heroin, or crack cocaine.

There are only a few basic characters used to represent numerical values in the Roman numeral system. These characters can be arranged to represent every number from 1 to 3999 using a standard set of rules.

I = 1

V = 5

X = 10

L = 50

C = 100

D = 500

M = 1000

Roman numerals are read left to right just like regular numbers. However, the letters of the Roman numerals are added together to identify the numbers in the ones, tens, hundreds, and thousands places. For example, the number 2 is represented by two "I" Roman numeral characters, so that "II" means "1 + 1" or the value of 2. The number 7 would be "VII" which would mean "5 + 1 + 1" for the value of 7. "XI" would be 11, and "CVI" would be "100 + 5 + 1" for a value of 106.

Notice how the organization of the Roman numerals just described is arranged left to right with the characters appearing in order of descending value. So, for CVI, the hundred symbol C is farthest left, the V symbol for 5 is next, and the I symbol for 1 is farthest right. "XXV" would be "10 + 10 + 5" with the value of 25, and LXVII would be "50 + 10 + 5 + 1 + 1" with the value of 67.

However, the exception to that rule would be numbers with 4 or 9 in them. Instead of the value 4 being represented as IIII (1 + 1 + 1 + 1) and the value of 9 being VIIII (5 + 1 + 1 + 1 + 1), the Roman numeral system uses "IV" for the value of 4 and "IX" for the value of 9. In these two cases, the lower value character ("I") comes *before* the higher value character ("V" or "X") when reading the Roman numeral left to right. When this happens, it signals that the smaller valued character is *subtracted* from the value of the number next to it on the right. Therefore, IV translates to "5 – 1" and has the value of 4, while IX translates to "10 – 1" and has the value of 9. The value of 29 would be XXIX (10 + 10 – 1 + 10 = 29) and XXXIV would be 34 (10 + 10 + 10 – 1 + 5 = 34).

Table 11.2 Examples of Roman numeral representation of numbers containing the digits 4 and 9

Value	Roman numeral
4	IV
14	XIV
40	XL
44	XLIV
400	CD
444	CDXLIV
9	IX
39	XXXIX
90	XC
99	XCIX
900	CM
949	CMXLIX
999	CMXCIX

These examples all have the 4 or 9 located in the ones place, but the same type of arrangement can occur using other Roman numeral characters in the tens, hundreds, or thousands place. For example, the value 40 would be XL (–10 + 50 = 40) and the value for 900 would be CM (–100 + 1000 = 900). So whenever there is a lower value Roman numeral character immediately to the left of a higher value character, you need "to subtract" its value. Table 11.2 shows some Roman numerals of numbers containing the digits 4 and 9.

Larger Roman numerals may appear daunting to read or write, but the characters used simply identify what number goes in the ones, tens, hundreds, etc. places. For example, MMCCCLXXIII is the value of 2373. Either the values of the individual characters can be added up, paying special attention to those situations where numbers 4 or 9 are represented by a lower character preceding a higher value character when read left to right, or the numbers in each column of ones, tens, etc. can be determined. Reading the Roman numeral MMCCCLXXIII from the left to the right, there are 2 "M" characters so the thousands place is occupied by a "2" giving the value of the Roman numeral 2000. Three "C" characters mean there is a "3" in the hundreds place, adding 300 to the value of the number. The tens place is a "7" for 70 as indicated by the "L" for 50 and the two "X" characters for 20. Finally, the ones place is a "3" for the "III". Putting the numbers in their places in order or adding up the values of the individual characters gives the total value of 2373.

For another more difficult example, try this one: MCMXLIV. A quick look over the characters identifies three pairs of characters that do not transition from higher value to lower value as they are read left to right: C to M is 100 to 1000, X to L is 10 to 50, and I to V is 1 to 5. Therefore, there are some values of characters that must be subtracted to determine the total value of the number.

- M is 1000 but CM is –100 + 1000 or 900. Thus, MCM is 1000 + 900, which is 1900.

- Now look at the next pair: XL is –10 + 50, which is 40. 40 added to the 1900 gives a value of 1940 so far.

- Finally, IV is –1 + 5, which is 4. When added to the value of the other characters, this gives the full value of the Roman numeral as 1944.

For values above 3999, the characters used previously are modified to represent values 5000 and higher. A bar over a Roman numeral character means it is 1000 times the character's normal value.

$$\bar{V} = 5 \times 1000 = 5000$$

$$\bar{X} = 10 \times 1000 = 10\,000$$

$$\bar{L} = 50 \times 1000 = 50\,000$$

$$\bar{C} = 100 \times 1000 = 100\,000$$

$$\bar{D} = 50 \times 1000 = 50\,000$$

$$I\bar{V} = 4 \times 1000 = 4000$$

$$I\bar{X} = 9 \times 1000 = 9000$$

These large-value Roman numerals are rarely used and this information has been provided simply to illustrate how number values of 4000 and above might be represented.

By practicing translating Roman numerals into numbers and vice versa, the veterinary professional can become familiar with the basic characters and quickly recognize the numeric values represented by strings of Roman numerals.

11.4 Chapter 11 Practice Problems

1 For each data set identify the mean, median, mode, and range:

A) 2, 4, 5, 6, 7, 9, 9, 11, 12, 15, 16
B) 23, 26, 32, 35, 36, 37, 37, 38, 38, 38, 39, 39, 40, 40, 41, 42, 44
C) 1.25, 1.29, 1.34, 1.36, 1.37, 1.38, 1.38, 1.38, 1.38, 1.39, 1.42
D) −2.4, −1.8, −0.5, −0.2, −0.1, 0.1, 0.2, 0.3, 0.3, 0.3, 0.4, 0.5, 0.7, 0.8
E) 32.3, 17.2, 22.3, 19.5, 20.6, 29.3, 22.3, 30.1, 24.4, 27.9, 25.4, 26.5

2 For each of the following Fahrenheit values, convert to Celsius (centigrade):

A) 60 °F
B) 90 °F
C) 104 °F
D) 108 °F
E) −9 °F
F) 101.5 °F
G) 99 °F
H) 128 °F
I) 102.4 °F
J) 100.8 °F

3 For each of the following Celsius (centigrade) values, convert to Fahrenheit:

A) 35 °C
B) 42 °C
C) 12 °C
D) −3 °C
E) 37 °C
F) 40.5 °C
G) −45 °C
H) 37.7 °C
I) 36.3 °C
J) 38.2 °C

4   Given the following Roman numerals, write the value for each:

A) XII
B) XXV
C) XLVII
D) LXIV
E) XCIII
F) CXXIX
G) CCCXXXIV
H) MCCXXXVII
I) MCMXXXV
J) MCMXCVIII

5   For each of the following values, write the corresponding Roman numerals:

A) 8
B) 23
C) 45
D) 102
E) 319
F) 477
G) 816
H) 1393
I) 1994
J) 2019

6   Given the following Roman numerals, write the value for each Roman numeral, solve the problem, and then write the solution to the problem in Roman numerals:

A) XIII + CXV = ???
B) XV + XLII = ???
C) XCV – XXIV = ???
D) CXIV – XLIX = ???
E) DCXIII + CDXIII = ???
F) XCIX + CI + LXXIV = ???
G) MMCCCXXVI – MCMXIX = ???
H) MLII – DI = ???

7   The medical record on the patient states that this patient had a body temperature of 38 °C yesterday. Today, the temperature registers 100.9 °F on your thermometer. Is the body temperature today higher, lower, or same as yesterday?

Appendix: Answers to Practice Problems

Chapter 1 Answers to Self-Assessment Exercises

1 For review of this section, see Chapter 2, Section 2.5.

A) 2.3×10 or 2.3×10^1

B) 1.32×10^2

C) 5.22178×10^5

D) 2×10^{-1}

E) 4.52×10^{-2}

F) 6.7×10^{-5}

G) 9.40023×10 or 9.40023×10^1

H) 8.9701×10^2

2 For review of this section, see Chapter 2, Sections 2.1, 2.2, 2.3, and 2.6.

A) 5.5

B) 11.6

C) 13.98

D) 0.51

E) 4.009

Medical Mathematics and Dosage Calculations for Veterinary Technicians, Third Edition. Robert Bill.
© 2019 John Wiley & Sons, Inc. Published 2019 by John Wiley & Sons, Inc.
Companion website: www.wiley.com/go/bill/calculations

F) 5

G) 5.1

H) 21.625

I) 0.456

J) 0.00262 or 2.62×10^{-3}

K) 1.99 mL

L) 333.2 g

M) 43.83 mg

N) 26.525 mL

3   For review of this section, see Chapter 2, Sections 2.1. 2.2, 2.3, and 2.7.

A) 12.5

B) 25.05

C) 305.6625

D) 0.31

E) 0.0000375 or 3.75×10^{-5}

F) 6

G) 1.667

H) 70

I) 2

J) 4

K) 30 mg

L) 150 mL

M) 216.2 mg

N) 40 mg

O) 11 mL

P) 14.25 mL

4 For review of this section, see Chapter 2, Sections 2.2 and 2.9.

1/100th	1/10th
A) 20.39	20.4
B) 9.68	9.7
C) 3.23	3.2
D) 29.45	29.5
E) 413.68	413.7
F) 5.96	6.0
G) 36.79	36.8
H) 0.26	0.3
I) 0.09	0.1
J) 1200.02	1200.0
K) 15.8 mg	
L) 38 mg; closer to 40 mg tablet size	

5 For review of this section, see Chapter 3, Sections 3.1, 3.2, 3.3, and 3.4.

A) $\dfrac{1}{5}$

B) $\dfrac{1}{4}$

C) $\dfrac{1}{4}$

D) $1\dfrac{3}{4}$

E) $5\dfrac{1}{8}$

6 For review of this section, see Chapter 3, Sections 3.5 and 3.6.

A) 1

B) $\dfrac{5}{32}$

C) $\dfrac{17}{30}$

D) $4\dfrac{1}{4}$

E) $10\dfrac{13}{24}$

F) $\dfrac{1}{4}$

G) $\dfrac{3}{6} = \dfrac{1}{2}$

H) $\dfrac{7}{8}$

I) $1\dfrac{9}{16}$

J) $11\dfrac{13}{40}$

7 For review of this section, see Chapter 3, Section 3.7.

A) $\dfrac{1}{4}$

B) $\dfrac{3}{8}$

C) $\dfrac{9}{16}$

D) $1\dfrac{5}{16}$

E) $\dfrac{33}{64}$

F) $12\dfrac{3}{8}$

G) $9\dfrac{3}{4}$

H) $96\dfrac{20}{24} = 96\dfrac{10}{12} = 96\dfrac{5}{6}$

8   For review of this section, see Chapter 3, Section 3.8.

A) 2

B) $\dfrac{2}{3}$

C) $\dfrac{18}{12} = \dfrac{3}{2} = 1\dfrac{1}{2}$

D) 8

E) 5

F) 60

G) 360

H) $782\dfrac{1}{2}$

9   For review of this section, see Chapter 3, Section 3.9.

A) 0.2

B) 0.5

C) 0.142857

D) 1.5

E) 4.833

F) 15.4375

10   For review of this section, see Chapter 3, Section 3.9.

A) $\dfrac{1}{4}$

B) $\dfrac{1}{3}$

C) $\dfrac{3}{4}$

D) $\dfrac{1}{8}$

E) $1\dfrac{1}{2}$

F) $2\dfrac{1}{2}$

11   For review of this section, see Chapter 4, Section 4.1.

A) $\dfrac{25}{100} = \dfrac{1}{4}$

B) $\dfrac{75}{100} = \dfrac{3}{4}$

C) $\dfrac{333}{1000} = \dfrac{1}{3}$

D) $\dfrac{10}{100} = \dfrac{1}{10}$

E) $\dfrac{80}{100} = \dfrac{8}{10} = \dfrac{4}{5}$

12   For review of this section, see Chapter 4, Section 4.2.

A) 0.25

B) 0.79

C) 1

D) 0.06

E) 0.002

F) 0.000087

13 For review of this section, see Chapter 4, Section 4.2.

   A) 50%

   B) 45%

   C) 100%

   D) 10.3%

   E) 90.023%

14 For review of this section, see Chapter 4, Section 4.3.

   A) 75%

   B) 80%

   C) 33.3%

   D) 1%

   E) 0.1%

15 For review of this section, see Chapter 4, Sections 4.4, 4.5, and 4.6.

   A) 50 mg

   B) 12.5 mg

   C) 20%

   D) 25%

16 For review of this section, see Chapter 5, Sections 5.1, 5.2, and 5.3.

   A) $X = 60$

   B) $X = 8$

   C) $X = 3.8$

   D) $X = 13$

   E) $X = 3.6$

   F) $X = 25.7$

17　For review of this section, see Chapter 5, Sections 5.4 and 5.7.

A) $X = 4$

B) $X = 8$

C) $X = 20.75$

D) $X = 2$

E) $X = 195$

F) $X = 16.67$

18　For review of this section, see Chapter 5, Sections 5.5, 5.6, and 5.8.

A) $X = 4$

B) $X = 12$

C) $X = 64$

D) $X = 36$

E) $X = 3$

Chapter 2 Answers

1　7

2　A) 25.69

B) 33 452.648 (note no use of commas, but there is a space between the thousands and the hundreds)

C) 367.2104

D) 0.026 (note the inclusion of zero in the ones place)

3　0.012 (make sure to put the zero in the ones place)

4　A) 12.30 cc

B) 0.25 g

C) 132.3 mL

D) 0.003 mg/mL

5 A) 342.00
   There are no trailing numbers after the decimal point. The exception would be if the answer required the answer to be precise to the nearest one hundredths place. The correct way to write the number would be 342.

   B) .653
   There is no zero in the ones place to call attention to the decimal point and the decimal point could be accidentally overlooked. It should be correctly written as 0.653.

   C) The zero between the integer 3 in the hundredths place and the decimal point was ignored. The way the person read the number would give the value of 7.38, not 7.038. The correct way to read the number would be "seven point zero three eight."

   D) When reading a decimal number in this fashion, the fractional part of the decimal number (the numbers to the right of the decimal point) is read using the decimal fraction place farthest to the right only. The correct way to read this number would be "three and twenty-five hundredths."

6 A) 0.1936

   B) 0.00521

   C) 0.5

   D) 0.0009

   E) 0.008

7 Add trailing zeroes to the end of 0.02 and 0.04 to produce the same number of digits in these numbers as 0.0033 and then compare the numbers. 0.02 becomes 0.0200 and 0.04 becomes 0.0400. These numbers have the same values as the original because the trailing zeroes do not alter the value. Comparing 0.0200 and 0.0400 to 0.0033, the range numbers look like 200 and 400 and the 0.0033 looks like just 33. 33 is outside of the acceptable range of 200–400, therefore this drug concentration of 0.0033 mcg/mL is below the acceptable range of 0.02–0.04 mcg/mL. This comparison is easier and the size relationship easier to see if all three numbers are "stacked" on top of each other with their decimal points aligned:

   0.0200

   0.0400

   0.0033

8 Add trailing zeroes to all numbers to produce equivalent numbers with the same number of digits. 0.012 becomes 0.0120, 0.02 becomes 0.0200, and 0.0075 keeps its same form. Stacking the numbers clearly shows that the 0.0120 mg/h drug rate is acceptably between 0.0200 and 0.0075 mg/h.

   0.0200

   0.0120

   0.0075

9   A) 3.673×10^3

    B) 2.35233×10^5

    C) 5.0×10^0 or 5×10

    D) 8.66×10^2

    E) 5.26303×10^3

    F) 7×10^{-1}

    G) 2.5×10^{-2}

    H) 4.304×10^{-4}

    I) 2.0×10^{-2}

    J) 7.5×10^{-6}

10 A) 240

    B) 16 670

    C) 539 010

    D) 10.03

    E) 6260.045

    F) 0.0832

    G) 0.000 010 05

    H) 0.000 009 012 403

11 A) 6.8

    B) 17.88

    C) 150.275

    D) 1.264

   E) 45.212 476

   F) 9.6

   G) 358.36

   H) 1.3433

   I) 0.262

   J) 12.034 25

12 A) 15.9

   B) 33

   C) 7.725

   D) 51.5

13 A) 25.41

   B) 50.4489

   C) 1.2145

   D) 0.029 13

   E) 21.876 081 = rounds to 21.876 = 21.88 = 21.9

14 A) 9

   B) 6.5

   C) 97.11

   D) 109.721 04 = rounds to 109.7210 = 109.721 = 109.72 = 109.7

   E) 726.363

   F) 170.573 202 = rounds to 170.5732 = 170.573 = 170.57 = 170.6

   G) 7.38

H) 1.23246 = rounds to 1.2325 = 1.233 = 1.23 = 1.2

I) 0.093 006 = rounds to 0.09301 = 0.0930 = 0.093 = 0.09 = 0.1

J) 0.796 26 = rounds to 0.7963 = 0.796 = 0.80 = 0.8

K) 0.0312 = rounds to 0.031 = 0.03

L) 156.110 004 = rounds to 156.110 00 = 156.1100 = 156.110 = 156.11 = 156.1

M) 3735.653 09 = rounds to 3735.6531 = 3735.653 = 3735.65 = 3735.7 = 3736

N) 0.514 971 = rounds to 0.514 97 = 0.5150 = 0.515 = 0.52 = 0.5

O) 88.542 076 = rounds to 88.54208 = 88.5421 = 88.542 = 88.54 = 88.5 = 89

P) 0.662 351 97 = rounds to 0.662 3520 = 0.662 352 = 0.662 35 = 0.6624 = 0.662 = 0.66 = 0.7

Q) 0.038 4651 = rounds to 0.038 4651 = 0.038 465 = 0.03847 = 0.0385 = 0.039 = 0.04

R) 1104.0021 = rounds to 1104.002 = 1104.00 = 1104.0 = 1104

S) 3.422 936 = rounds to 3.422 94 = 3.4229 = 3.423 = 3.43 = 3.4 = 3

T) 0.000 0392 = rounds to 0.000 039 = 0.000 04 = 4×10^{-5}

15 A) 2.1

B) 0.015 625 = rounds to 0.01563 = 0.0156 = 0.016 = 0.02

C) 12.3

D) 2.007 843 14 = rounds to 2.007 8431 = 2.007 843 = 2.007 84 = 2.0078 = 2.008 = 2.01 = 2

E) 37.439 442 92 = rounds to 37.439 4430 = 3.439 44 = 3.4394 = 3.439 = 3.44 = 3.4

F) 6.062 1212 (repeating) = rounds to 6.062 12 = 6.0621 = 6.062 = 6.06 = 6.1

16 A) 11.1

B) 35

C) 71.856 287 43 = rounds to 71.856 2874 = 71.856 287 = 71.856 29 = 71.8563 = 71.856 = 71.86 = 71.9

D) 593.391 836 61 = rounds to 593.391 8366 = 593.391 837 = 593.391 84 = 593.3918 = 593.392 = 593.4

E) 6.666 (repeating) = rounds to 6.667 = 6.67 = 6.7

F) 7.425 997 43 = rounds to 7.425 9974 = 7.425 997 = 7.426 00 = 7.426 = 7.43 = 7.4

G) 2.977 325 65 = rounds to 2.977 3257 = 2.977 326 = 2.977 33 = 2.9773 = 2.977 = 3.00 = 3

H) 0.274 316 94 = rounds to 0.274 3169 = 0.274 317 = 0.27432 = 0.2743 = 0.274 = 0.27 = 0.3

I) 0.009 6217 = rounds to 0.009 622 = 0.009 62 = 0.0096 = 0.010 = 1×10^{-2}

J) 100.379 734 85 = rounds to 100.379 7349 = 100.379 735 = 100.379 74 = 100.3797 = 100.380 = 100.4

17 A) 220

B) 1540

C) 12

18 A) 32.1

B) 1.17

C) 9

D) 4000

E) 41.0

F) 800

G) 0.33

H) 9.94

I) 0.001

J) 0.0093

K) 0.014 264

L) 2.1928

M) 5.556

19 A) 0.134 615 38 rounds to 0.13

B) 2.0196 rounds to 2.02

Chapter 3 Answers

1 A) True

B) False

C) True

D) True

E) False

F) True

2 A) $\dfrac{1}{2} = \dfrac{2}{4} = \dfrac{8}{16} = \dfrac{50}{100}$

B) $\dfrac{1}{3} = \dfrac{4}{12} = \dfrac{11}{33} = \dfrac{41}{123}$

C) $\dfrac{2}{5} = \dfrac{6}{15} = \dfrac{22}{55} = \dfrac{100}{250}$

D) $\dfrac{7}{8} = \dfrac{56}{64} = \dfrac{84}{96} = \dfrac{280}{320}$

E) $2\dfrac{13}{16} = 2\dfrac{52}{64} = 2\dfrac{390}{480} = 2\dfrac{2925}{3600}$

3 A) $\dfrac{4}{10} = \dfrac{2}{5}$

B) $\dfrac{6}{16} = \dfrac{3}{8}$

C) $\dfrac{24}{36} = \dfrac{2}{3}$

D) $\dfrac{36}{42} = \dfrac{18}{21}$

E) $\dfrac{72}{12} = \dfrac{6}{1} = 6$

F) $\dfrac{73}{1} = 73$

G) $2\dfrac{4}{8} = 2\dfrac{1}{2}$

H) $5\dfrac{24}{16} = 5\dfrac{3}{2} = 6\dfrac{1}{2}$

4 A) $\dfrac{8}{100}\,\text{g} = \dfrac{2}{25}\,\text{g}$

B) $\dfrac{45}{125}\,\text{kg} = \dfrac{9}{25}\,\text{kg}$

C) $\dfrac{56}{128}\,\text{kg} = \dfrac{7}{16}\,\text{kg}$

D) $\dfrac{512}{768}\,\text{L} = \dfrac{128}{192}\,\text{L}$

E) $\dfrac{19}{57}\,\text{g} = \dfrac{1}{3}\,\text{g}$

5 A) $\dfrac{2}{8} + \dfrac{3}{8} = \dfrac{5}{8}$

B) $\dfrac{3}{6} + \dfrac{6}{18} = \dfrac{15}{18} = \dfrac{5}{6}$

C) $\dfrac{4}{48} + \dfrac{23}{24} = \dfrac{50}{48} = \dfrac{25}{24} = 1\dfrac{1}{24}$

D) $\dfrac{3}{14} + \dfrac{35}{56} = \dfrac{47}{56}$

E) $\dfrac{4}{12} + \dfrac{7}{36} = \dfrac{19}{36}$

F) $\dfrac{32}{16} + \dfrac{14}{28} = \dfrac{2}{1} + \dfrac{1}{2} = 2\dfrac{1}{2}$

G) $1\dfrac{3}{5} + \dfrac{49}{10} = 1\dfrac{55}{10} = 6\dfrac{5}{10} = 6\dfrac{1}{2}$

H) $3\dfrac{14}{8} + 5\dfrac{24}{5} = 4\dfrac{6}{8} + 9\dfrac{4}{5} = 4\dfrac{3}{4} + 9\dfrac{4}{5} = 13\dfrac{31}{20} = 14\dfrac{11}{20}$

I) $\dfrac{13}{8} + 4 + \dfrac{8}{24} = \dfrac{39}{24} + 4 + \dfrac{8}{24} = 5\dfrac{23}{24}$

J) $1\dfrac{1}{2} + 3\dfrac{3}{4} + 12\dfrac{7}{8} + \dfrac{24}{36} = \dfrac{3}{2} + \dfrac{15}{4} + \dfrac{103}{8} + \dfrac{2}{3} = \dfrac{36}{24} + \dfrac{90}{24} + \dfrac{309}{24} + \dfrac{16}{24} = 18\dfrac{19}{24}$

6   A) $\dfrac{8}{16} - \dfrac{5}{16} = \dfrac{3}{16}$

B) $\dfrac{4}{10} - \dfrac{7}{40} = \dfrac{9}{40}$

C) $\dfrac{14}{28} - \dfrac{3}{14} = \dfrac{8}{28} = \dfrac{4}{14}$

D) $\dfrac{43}{12} - \dfrac{31}{18} = \dfrac{774}{216} - \dfrac{372}{216} = \dfrac{402}{216} = \dfrac{201}{108} = \dfrac{67}{36} = 1\dfrac{31}{36}$

E) $\dfrac{32}{64} - \dfrac{45}{128} = \dfrac{1}{2} - \dfrac{45}{128} = \dfrac{64}{128} - \dfrac{45}{128} = \dfrac{19}{128}$

F) $2\dfrac{3}{6} - 1\dfrac{8}{24} = 2\dfrac{3}{6} - 1\dfrac{2}{6} = \dfrac{15}{6} - \dfrac{8}{6} = \dfrac{7}{6} = 1\dfrac{1}{6}$

G) $8\dfrac{1}{4} - 5\dfrac{3}{4} = \dfrac{33}{4} - \dfrac{23}{4} = \dfrac{10}{4} = 2\dfrac{2}{4} = 2\dfrac{1}{2}$

H) $12\dfrac{1}{2} - 9\dfrac{3}{4} = \dfrac{25}{2} - \dfrac{39}{4} = \dfrac{50}{4} - \dfrac{39}{4} = \dfrac{11}{4} = 2\dfrac{3}{4}$

I) $\dfrac{38}{12} - 1\dfrac{14}{8} = \dfrac{38}{12} - \dfrac{22}{8} = \dfrac{76}{24} - \dfrac{66}{24} = \dfrac{10}{24} = \dfrac{5}{12}$

J) $3\dfrac{12}{8} - 1\dfrac{2}{12} = \dfrac{36}{8} - \dfrac{14}{12} = \dfrac{108}{24} - \dfrac{28}{24} = \dfrac{80}{24} = \dfrac{10}{3} = 3\dfrac{1}{3}$

7   A) $\dfrac{1}{4} \times \dfrac{1}{2} = \dfrac{1}{8}$

B) $\dfrac{3}{8} \times \dfrac{5}{6} = \dfrac{15}{48} = \dfrac{5}{16}$

C) $\dfrac{32}{3} \times \dfrac{3}{5} = \dfrac{32}{5} = 6\dfrac{2}{5}$

D) $\dfrac{2}{5} \times \dfrac{16}{10} = \dfrac{16}{25}$

E) $\dfrac{14}{4} \times \dfrac{26}{12} = \dfrac{91}{12} = 7\dfrac{7}{12}$

F) $5 \times \dfrac{5}{6} = 4\dfrac{1}{6}$

G) $\dfrac{32}{18} \times 4 = \dfrac{64}{9} = 7\dfrac{1}{9}$

H) $2\dfrac{2}{3} \times 4\dfrac{5}{6} = \dfrac{8}{3} \times \dfrac{29}{6} = \dfrac{116}{9} = 12\dfrac{8}{9}$

I) $1\dfrac{1}{2} \times 3\dfrac{3}{4} = \dfrac{3}{2} \times \dfrac{15}{4} = \dfrac{45}{8} = 5\dfrac{5}{8} =$

J) $12\dfrac{1}{4} \times 24\dfrac{1}{2} \times 4\dfrac{3}{4} = \dfrac{49}{4} \times \dfrac{49}{2} \times \dfrac{19}{4} = \dfrac{45619}{32} = 1425\dfrac{19}{32}$

8 A) $\dfrac{1}{2} \div \dfrac{3}{4} = \dfrac{1}{2} \times \dfrac{4}{3} = \dfrac{2}{3}$

B) $\dfrac{4}{5} \div \dfrac{1}{5} = \dfrac{4}{5} \times \dfrac{5}{1} = \dfrac{4}{1} = 4$

C) $\dfrac{3}{8} \div 2 = \dfrac{3}{8} \times \dfrac{1}{2} = \dfrac{3}{16}$

D) $\dfrac{16}{32} \div \dfrac{2}{8} = \dfrac{16}{32} \times \dfrac{8}{2} = \dfrac{16}{4} \times \dfrac{1}{2} = \dfrac{16}{8} = 2$

E) $1\dfrac{1}{2} \div \dfrac{3}{8} = \dfrac{3}{2} \times \dfrac{8}{3} = 4$

F) $3\dfrac{1}{4} \div 8 = \dfrac{13}{4} \times \dfrac{1}{8} = \dfrac{13}{32}$

G) $12\dfrac{3}{16} \div 2\dfrac{1}{8} = \dfrac{195}{16} \times \dfrac{8}{17} = \dfrac{195}{2} \times \dfrac{1}{17} = \dfrac{195}{34} = 5\dfrac{25}{34}$

H) $39\dfrac{12}{32} \div 5\dfrac{14}{16} = \dfrac{1260}{32} \times \dfrac{16}{94} = \dfrac{1260}{2} \times \dfrac{1}{94} = \dfrac{1260}{188} = \dfrac{315}{47} = 6\dfrac{33}{47}$

I) $342\dfrac{12}{16} \div 23\dfrac{34}{64} = \dfrac{5484}{16} \times \dfrac{64}{1506} = \dfrac{5484}{1} \times \dfrac{4}{1506} = \dfrac{21936}{1506} = 14\dfrac{852}{1506} = 14\dfrac{426}{753}$

J) $\dfrac{125}{15} \div 7\dfrac{8}{50} = \dfrac{125}{15} \times \dfrac{50}{358} = \dfrac{25}{3} \times \dfrac{25}{179} = \dfrac{625}{537} = 1\dfrac{88}{537}$

9 A) $\dfrac{3}{4} = 0.75$

B) $\dfrac{9}{10} = 0.9$

C) $\dfrac{7}{8} = 0.875$

D) $\dfrac{23}{35} = 0.657\,143$

E) $\dfrac{48}{16} = 3$

F) $\dfrac{39}{24} = 1.625$

G) $2\dfrac{3}{4} = 2.75$

H) $23\dfrac{13}{32} = 23.406\,25$

I) $45\dfrac{15}{18} = 45.8333\overline{3}$

J) $231\dfrac{81}{125} = 231.648$

10 A) $\dfrac{1}{2}$ tablet

B) $1\dfrac{3}{4}$ tablets

C) 3 tablets

D) $12\dfrac{3}{4}$ tablets

E) $5\dfrac{3}{4}$ tablets

11 A) $\dfrac{7}{16} = \dfrac{1}{2}$

   B) $\dfrac{17}{64} = \dfrac{1}{4}$

   C) $\dfrac{23}{5} = 4\dfrac{1}{2}$

   D) $6\dfrac{2}{3} = 6\dfrac{3}{4}$

   E) $23\dfrac{17}{32} = 23\dfrac{1}{2}$

12 A) Days 1–3 (3 days) = 1.5 tablets 2× daily for 3 days = 1.5 × 2 × 3 = 9 tablets

   B) Days 4–6 (3 days) = 1 tablet 1× daily for 3 days = 1 × 1 × 3 = 3 tablets

   C) Days 7–9 (3 days) = 0.75 tablet 1× daily for 3 days = 0.75 × 1 × 3 = 2.25 tablets

   D) Days 10–14 (5 days) = 0.25 tablet 1× daily for 5 days = 0.25 × 1 × 5 = 1.25
      Total tablets = 9 + 3 + 2.25 + 1.25 = 15.5 tablets needed.
      16 whole tablets dispensed.

13 36 mg × 0.5 = 18 mg in the adjusted dose.

   18 mg + 3.75 mg = 21.75 mg to compensate for drug stuck to IV set

   21.75 mg – 1.825 mg = 19.925 mg for final calculated dose.

Chapter 4 Answers

1 A) 0.5

   B) 0.25

   C) 0.015

   D) 0.007

   E) 0.1023

   F) 0.00085

G) 1.25

H) 2.0355

2   A) 75%

B) 12.5%

C) 1.5%

D) 0.35%

E) 10%

F) 8.125%

G) 125%

H) 300.1%

3   A) $\dfrac{1}{2}$

B) $\dfrac{1}{4}$

C) $\dfrac{1}{8}$

D) $\dfrac{1}{100}$

E) $\dfrac{1}{1000}$

F) $\dfrac{1}{4000}$

G) $1\dfrac{1}{4}$

H) $5\dfrac{1}{8}$

4   A) 50%

B) 75%

    C) 12.5%

    D) 3.125%

    E) 10%

    F) 40%

    G) 28.125%

    H) 42.86%

5   1.25 or the dose can multiplied by 0.25 and that amount added back to the original.

6   33%

7   25%

8   25 mg (250 mg × 0.1 = 25 mg)

9   30 mg (200 mg × 0.15 = 30 mg)

    170 mg (200 mg − 30 mg = 170 mg)

10 90 mg (120 mg × 0.25 = 30 mg; 120 mg − 30 mg = 90 mg; or 120 mg ×0.75 = 90 mg)

11 50% decrease

12 300% increase

13 reduced by 87.5% (2000 − 250 = 1750; 1750/2000 = 0.875 = 87.5%); 12.5% of original is left.

14 3 mL are left; 27 mL have been removed

15 2 × X mg = current dose

16 525 mg (600 mg × 12.5% = 600 mg × 0.125 = 75 mg; 600 mg − 75 mg = 525 mg)

17 105 mg (175% = 1.75; 1.75 × 60 mg = 105 mg)

18 A) 0.25 × 600 mg = 150 mg

    B) 0.45 × 300 mg = 135 mg

    C) 0.75 × 200 mg = 150 mg

    D) 2.00×50 mg = 100 mg

    E) $12.5 \div 37.5$ (12.5/37.5) = 0.333 = 33.3%

    F) 0.25×200 mg = 50 mg amount added 200 mg + 50 mg = 250 mg new dose

Chapter 5 Answers

1 A) 15

    B) 317.6

    C) 0.2724

    D) 39.5

    E) $62\dfrac{2}{6} = 62\dfrac{1}{3} = 62.33\bar{3}$

    F) 50 mL (must include mL units)

    G) 68 mg

    H) 6.17 L

    I) 0.027 g

    J) $-\dfrac{9}{12} = -\dfrac{3}{4} = -0.75\,\text{kg}$

2 A) 17

    B) 345

    C) −0.5

    D) $33\dfrac{3}{6} = 33\dfrac{1}{2} = 33.5$

    E) $\dfrac{5}{12} = 0.41666\bar{6} = 0.4167\,\text{rounded}$

    F) 75 gr

    G) 57 mg

H) 67.5 gr

I) 0.0113 mcg

J) $\dfrac{5}{24} = 0.208\,33\bar{3}\,\text{kg}$

3 A) 5

B) 1.7559

C) $\dfrac{3}{7} = 0.428\,57$

D) $\dfrac{40}{63} = 0.634\,921$

E) $\dfrac{52}{45} = 1\dfrac{7}{45} = 1.155\bar{5} = 1.156\,\text{rounded}$

F) $\dfrac{80}{144} = \dfrac{20}{36} = \dfrac{5}{9} = 0.555\bar{5} = 0.556\,\text{rounded}$

G) $\dfrac{65}{624} = 0.104\,166\bar{6} = 0.104\,167\,\text{rounded}$

H) $\dfrac{380}{366} = \dfrac{190}{183} = 1.038\,25$

I) 0.103 35

J) $-0.8888\bar{8} = -0.889\,\text{rounded}$

4 A) 5.881

B) 37.0414

C) 0.0103

D) 9.9017

E) $\dfrac{15}{16} = 0.9375$

F) $1\dfrac{1}{3} = 1.33\bar{3}$

G) $\dfrac{1}{6} = 0.166\bar{6} = 0.1667$ rounded

H) $\dfrac{2}{3} = 0.666\bar{6} = 0.6667$ rounded

I) $6\dfrac{1}{8} = 6.125$

J) $0.0755\bar{5} = 0.0756$ rounded

5   3 mL + 12 mL = 5.75 mL + X mL; X = 9.25 mL

6    $360\,\text{mg} \times X = 240\,\text{mg}; X = \dfrac{240\,\text{mg}}{360\,\text{mg}}; X = \dfrac{2}{3}$ of a vial

7   45 mg + 7.5 mg = 30 mg + X mg; X = 22.5 mg

Chapter 6 Answers

1   A)   20 kg

    B)   10.3 mL

    C)   35 cc

    D)   5.1 mg

    E)   34.02 g (not 34.2 would be 34 and 2 tenths)

    F)   26.043 L

    G)   15 mg/kg

    H)   0.014 g/L

    I)   1.25 mcm or 1.25 μm

    J)   0.5 gr (g = grams, gr = grains)

    K)   20 lb

    L)   35 tsp

    M)   5.5 Tbsp

N) 3.25 fl oz

O) 6.25 c (1/4 = 0.25)

P) 15 gal

Q) 0.5 qt

2   A) 0.34 g

B) 325 g = 325 000 mg

C) 52 cc = 0.052 L

D) 25.1 mL

E) 3000 m

F) 400 mm = 0.4 m

G) 35.5 cm

H) 2500 m

I) 300 mg

J) 387.6 cm = 3.876 m

3   A) 25 kg

B) 2 kg

C) 44 lb

D) 20 mL = 0.02 L

E) 370 mL = 0.37 L

F) 18 tsp = 6 Tbsp

G) 1.5 gr = 0.09 g (60 mg = 1 grain conversion used)

H) 600 g = 10 000 gr = 1.32 lb

4   $0.25\,gr \times \dfrac{60\,mg}{1\,gr} = 15\,mg;\ \dfrac{15\,mg}{dose} \times \dfrac{2\,doses}{day} = \dfrac{30\,mg}{day} = 30\,mg\,a\,day$

5 $3\,\text{tsp} \times \dfrac{5\,\text{mL}}{1\,\text{tsp}} = 15\,\text{mL} = 15\,\text{cc}$; $15\,\text{cc} \times \dfrac{1\,\text{syringe}}{3\,\text{cc}} = 5\,\text{syringes}$

6 $850\,\text{lb} \times \dfrac{1\,\text{kg}}{2.2\,\text{lb}} = 386\,\text{kg}$

7 $100\,\text{mg} \times \dfrac{1\,\text{g}}{1000\,\text{mg}} = 0.1\,\text{g}$;

   $0.1\,\text{g} \times \dfrac{1\,\text{kg}}{1000\,\text{g}} = 0.0001\,\text{kg}$

   100 mg of additive per kilogram (the concentration in the new container) is NOT equivalent to 0.1 kg per kilogram (the concentration from the other manufacturer).

8 $\dfrac{0.5\,\text{gr}}{\text{tablet}} \times \dfrac{60\,\text{mg}}{1\,\text{gr}} = \dfrac{30\,\text{mg}}{\text{tablet}}$; $15\,\text{tablets} \times \dfrac{30\,\text{mg}}{\text{tablet}} = 450\,\text{mg total drug ingested}$

   $450\,\text{mg} \times \dfrac{1\,\text{g}}{1000\,\text{mg}} = 0.45\,\text{g}$; total ingested dose is below toxic dose.

9 $4.5\,\text{kg} \times \dfrac{2.2\,\text{lb}}{1\,\text{kg}} = 9.9\,\text{lb}$ or $4.5\,\text{lb} \times \dfrac{1\,\text{kg}}{2.2\,\text{lb}} = 2\,\text{kg}$

   A dose calculated for a 4.5 kg dog would be sufficient for a 9.9 lb dog and hence would be an overdose if given to a dog that weighs only 4.5 pounds.

10 $140\,\text{lb} \times \dfrac{1\,\text{kg}}{2.2\,\text{lb}} = 63.6\,\text{kg}$

   63.6 kg of animal body weight can be sedated with 35 mg of the drug.

   63.6 kg − 23 kg (Sam) − 10 kg (Bert) − 16.5 kg (Lilly) − 2.7 kg (Zamphire) − 4.3 kg (Ignatz) − 5.1 kg (Poindexter) leaves only enough drug to sedate an animal 2 kg or less. The next animal to be sedated (Shubert) needs enough drug to sedate his 4.2 kg body and hence there is not enough drug left over to administer a full dose to him.

11 A) estimate: 20 + 20 + 40 + 60 = 140; actual answer = 143

    B) estimate: 120 + 3500 + 900 + 40 = 4560; actual answer = 4571

    C) estimate: 46 − 32 = 14, which (×10) would be 140; actual answer = 139

    D) estimate: 90 − 49 = 41, which (×10) would be 410; actual answer = 403

    E) estimate: 3 × 6 = 18, which (×10, ×10) would be 1800; actual answer = 1830

    F) estimate: 100 × 50 = 5000; actual answer = 5390

    G) estimate: 48 divided by 6 = 8, which (×10) would be 80; actual answer = 80.83

Chapter 7 Answers

1 A) drug = diphenhydramine; dose = 50 mg; dose interval = 3 times a day; route = by mouth

   B) drug = ampicillin; dose = 300 mg; dose interval = every 12 hours; route = subcutaneously

2 A) q6h = q.i.d.

   B) t.i.d. = q 8 h

   C) EOD = q 2 d

   D) q.i.d. = q 6 h

   E) q12h = b.i.d.

3 A) Give one 50 mg amoxicillin tablet every eight hours by mouth.

   B) Give 125 grains of aspirin by mouth as needed.

   C) Give one 15 mg acepromazine tablet by mouth twice daily as needed.

   D) Apply neomycin ointment in both ears every four hours for seven days.

   E) Give 2 drops of tobramycin ophthalmic drops into the right eye every two hours.

   F) Give 20 mg of methylprednisolone subcutaneously every 2 days for 10 days.

   G) Give 120 mg of ampicillin intramuscularly.

   H) Give 30 grains of phenobarbital elixir every day by mouth.

4 A) Dermamaxx

   B) deracoxib

   C) deracoxib

   D) 100 mg

   E) Not a controlled substance. No "C" with a Roman numeral.

   F) Prescription drug. It contains the "legend" phrase restricting the "drug to use by or on the order of a licensed veterinarian."

5 A) No. There is no ® or TM to indicate a proprietary name owned by one company.

  B) cephalexin

  C) United States Pharmacopeia – a standard setting organization for manufacturing of drugs to be marketed in the United States

  D) No. There is a ℞ symbol on the label, indicating it is for prescription use only.

  E) No. There is no "C" with a Roman numeral.

6. A) 5% = 5 g/100 mL

  B) 0.3% = 0.3 g/100 mL

  C) 7.25% = 7.25 g/100 mL = 72.5 mg/mL

  D) 21.7% = 21.7 g/100 mL = 217 mg/mL

  E) 0.02% = 0.02 g/100 mL = 0.2 mg/mL

Chapter 8 Answers

1 A) 66 lb

  B) 40 kg

  C) 51.26 lb

  D) 612.73 kg

  E) 523.6 lb

  F) 10 kg

  G) 220 lb

  H) 359.8 kg

  I) 0.88 lb

  J) 0.386 kg

  K) 0.071 lb

L) 0.0145 kg

M) 3.092 kg

N) 11.64 lb

2 A) 86 mg

B) 10 mg

C) 693 mg

D) 25 mg

E) 815 mg

F) 0.125 mg

G) 193.2 mg

H) 195 mg

I) 98.2 mg

J) 82.5 mg

K) 0.26 mg

L) 1.0 mg

M) 0.9 mg

N) 1.8 mg

3 A) minimum 96.8 mg; maximum 242 mg

B) minimum 220 mg; maximum 275 mg

C) minimum 2727.3 mg; maximum 5454.5 mg

D) minimum 34.5 mg; maximum 57.5 mg

E) minimum 8.3 mg; maximum 16.5 mg

F) minimum 3300 mg; maximum 33 000 mg

G) minimum 6000 mg; maximum 9600 mg

4 A) 1.523 tablets; round to 1.5 tablets

B) 4.18 tablets; round to 4 tablets

C) 1.64 tablets; round to 1.5 tablets

D) 1.21 tablets; round to 1 tablet

E) 3.2 tablets; round to 3 tablets

F) 8.52 tablets; round to 8.5 tablets

G) 2.97 tablets; round to 3 tablets

H) 0.52 tablets; round to 0.5 tablet

5 A) 7.27 mL; round to 7.3 mL

B) 6.16 mL; round to 6.2 mL

C) 2.84 mL; round to 2.8 mL

D) 4.4 mL

E) 5.28 mL; round to 5.3 mL

F) 1.181 mL; round to 1.2 mL

G) 5.87 mL; round to 5.9 mL

H) 0.24 mL; round to 0.2 mL

6 A) 2.0 mL

B) 6.95 mL; round to 7.0 mL

C) 4.95 mL; round to 5.0 mL

D) 3.52 mL; round to 3.5 mL

E) 2.126 mL; round to 2.1 mL

7   A) 1 tablet/dose × 3 doses/day × 10 days = 30 tablets

    B) 2.068 tablet/dose; 2 tablets/dose × 2 doses/day × 5 days = 20 tablets

    C) 0.91 tablet/dose; 1 tablet/dose × 1 dose/day × 10 days = 10 tablets

    D) 0.836 tablet/dose; 1 tablet/dose × 2 dose/day × 12 days = 24 tablets

    E) 2.20 tablets/dose; 2 tablets/dose × 2 doses/day × 5 days = 20 tablets

    F) 4.125 tablets/dose; 4 tablets/dose × 2 doses/day × 7 days = 56 tablets

    G) 2.47 tablets/dose; 2.5 tablets/dose × 4 doses/day × 5 days = 50 tablets

    H) (1/2 grain = 30 mg) 1.424 tablets/dose; 1.5 tablet/dose × 1 dose/day × 180 days = 270 tablets

8   A) 0.5 cc or 0.5 mL

    B) 1.3 cc or 1.3 mL

    C) 2.0 cc or 2.0 mL

    D) 3.4 cc or 3.4 mL (note each mark is 0.2 mL)

    E) 15 cc or 15 mL

    F) 27 cc or 27 mL

9   A) Minimum dose = $125 \, \text{lb} \times \dfrac{\text{kg}}{2.2 \, \text{lb}} \times 20 \, \text{mg/kg} = 1136.4 \, \text{mg}$

        Maximum dose = $125 \, \text{lb} \times \dfrac{\text{kg}}{2.2 \, \text{lb}} \times 25 \, \text{mg/kg} = 1420.5 \, \text{mg}$

    B) Minimum volume = $1136.4 \, \text{mg} \times \dfrac{1 \, \text{mL}}{250 \, \text{mg}} = 4.545 \, \text{mL}$; 4.5 mL

        Maximum volume = $1420.5 \, \text{mg} \times \dfrac{1 \, \text{mL}}{250 \, \text{mg}} = 5.681 \, \text{mL}$; 5.7 mL

    C) $267/48 \, \text{mL} = \$5.56/\text{mL}$ or \$5.56 per mL

    D) Minimum dose cost = 4.5 mL/dose × \$5.56/mL = \$25.02 per dose
        Maximum dose cost = 5.7 mL/dose × \$5.56/mL = \$31.69 per dose

    E) Days for minimum dose = $48 \, \text{mL/vial} \times \dfrac{1 \, \text{day}}{4.5 \, \text{mL}} = 10.67 \, \text{days}$; 10 full days

        Days for maximum dose = $48 \, \text{mL/vial} \times \dfrac{1 \, \text{day}}{5.7 \, \text{mL}} = 8.42 \, \text{days}$; 8 full days

10 A) Jacquie, minimum dose = $13 \, \text{lb} \times \dfrac{1 \, \text{kg}}{2.2 \, \text{lb}} \times 5 \, \text{mg/kg} = 29.5 \, \text{mg}$

Jacquie, maximum dose = $13 \, \text{lb} \times \dfrac{1 \, \text{kg}}{2.2 \, \text{lb}} \times 10 \, \text{mg/kg} = 59.1 \, \text{mg}$

Jocko, minimum dose = $38 \, \text{lb} \times \dfrac{1 \, \text{kg}}{2.2 \, \text{lb}} \times 5 \, \text{mg/kg} = 86.4 \, \text{mg}$

Jocko, maximum dose = $38 \, \text{lb} \times \dfrac{1 \, \text{kg}}{2.2 \, \text{lb}} \times 10 \, \text{mg/kg} = 172.7 \, \text{mg}$

B) Jacquie, minimum tablet dose = 29.5 mg × 1 tablet/100 mg = 0.295 tablet, which rounds to 0.5 tablet
Jacquie, maximum tablet dose = 59.1 mg × 1 tablet/100 mg = 0.591 tablet, which rounds to 0.5 tablet
Jacquie should get 0.5 tablet per dose

Jocko, minimum tablet dose = $86.4 \times \dfrac{1 \, \text{tablet}}{100 \, \text{mg}} = 0.864$ tablet which rounds to 1.0 tablet

Jocko, maximum tablet dose = $172.7 \times \dfrac{1 \, \text{tablet}}{100 \, \text{mg}} = 1.727$ tablet which rounds to 1.5 tablet

Jocko could get either 1.0 tablet or 1.5 tablet depending upon the severity of his skin infection.

C) Jacquie total cost = 0.5 tablet/dose × 1 dose/day × 10 days = 5 tablets

11 A) 30 lb dog, minimum = $30 \, \text{lb} \times \dfrac{1 \, \text{kg}}{2.2 \, \text{lb}} \times 0.55 \, \text{mg/kg} = 7.5 \, \text{mg}$

30 lb dog, maximum = $30 \, \text{lb} \times \dfrac{1 \, \text{kg}}{2.2 \, \text{lb}} \times 2.2 \, \text{mg/kg} = 30 \, \text{mg}$

45 lb dog, minimum = $45 \, \text{lb} \times \dfrac{1 \, \text{kg}}{2.2 \, \text{lb}} \times 0.55 \, \text{mg/kg} = 11.25 \, \text{mg}$

45 lb dog, maximum = $45 \, \text{lb} \times \dfrac{1 \, \text{kg}}{2.2 \, \text{lb}} \times 2.2 \, \text{mg/kg} = 45 \, \text{mg}$

85 lb dog, minimum = $85 \, \text{lb} \times \dfrac{1 \, \text{kg}}{2.2 \, \text{lb}} \times 0.55 \, \text{mg/kg} = 21.25 \, \text{mg}$

85 lb dog, maximum = $85 \, \text{lb} \times \dfrac{1 \, \text{kg}}{2.2 \, \text{lb}} \times 2.2 \, \text{mg/kg} = 85 \, \text{mg}$

B) 30 lb dog, minimum tablets = $7.5 \, \text{mg} \times \dfrac{1 \, \text{tablet}}{25 \, \text{mg}} = 0.3$ tablet

30 lb dog, maximum tablets = $30 \, \text{mg} \times \dfrac{1 \, \text{tablet}}{25 \, \text{mg}} = 1.2$ tablet

Tablets cannot be split and the tablet dose must be within the minimum to maximum doses, so the only whole-tablet dose would be 1 tablet.

45 lb dog, minimum tablets = $11.25 \, \text{mg} \times \dfrac{1 \, \text{tablet}}{25 \, \text{mg}} = 0.45$ tablet

45 lb dog, maximum tablets = $45 \, \text{mg} \times \dfrac{1 \, \text{tablet}}{25 \, \text{mg}} = 1.8$ tablet

Tablets cannot be split and the tablet dose must be within the minimum to maximum doses, so the only whole-tablet dose would be 1 tablet. The dose cannot be rounded up to 2 tablets because that would be outside of the calculated dosage range.

85 lb dog, minimum tablets = 21.25 mg × 1 tablet/25 mg = 0.85 tablet

85 lb dog, maximum tablets = 85 mg × 1 tablet/25 mg = 3.4 tablet

Tablets cannot be split and the tablet dose must be within the minimum to maximum doses, so the best doses could be 1, 2, or 3 tablets as needed.

C) 30 lb dog = 4 doses × 1 tablet/dose × $0.75/tablet = $3.00 plus $8.00 dispensing fee = $11.00

45 lb dog = 4 doses × 1 tablet/dose × $0.75/tablet = $3.00 plus $8.00 dispensing fee = $11.00

85 lb dog = 4 doses × 3 tablet/dose × $0.75/tablet = $9.00 plus $8.00 dispensing fee = $17.00

Total cost for all medication = $39.00

Chapter 9 Answers

1 A) 2 mL/min

   B) 20 mL/min

   C) 16 mL/min

   D) 21 mL/min

   E) 6 mL/min

   F) 3 mL/min

   G) 2 mL/min

   H) 1.5 mL/min

   I) 6 mL/min

   J) 2 mL/min

2 A) 180 mL

   B) 30 mL

   C) 10 mL

   D) 40 mL

   E) 14.4 mL

   F) 72 mL

G) 112 mL

H) 36 mL

I) 1848 mL or 1.848 L

J) 960 mL

3   A)   45 gtt/min = 0.75 gtt/s = 15 drips every 20 seconds or 3 drips every 4 seconds

    B)   15 gtt/min = 0.25 gtt/s = 5 drips every 20 seconds or 1 drip every 4 seconds

    C)   48 gtt/min = 0.8 gtt/s = 8 drips every 10 seconds or 4 drips every 5 seconds

    D)   9 gtt/min = 0.15 gtt/s = 3 drips every 20 seconds

    E)   75 gtt/min = 1.25 gtt/s = 20 drips every 25 seconds or 5 drips every 4 seconds

    F)   100 gtt/min = 1.667 gtt/s = 25 drips every 15 seconds or 5 drips every 3 seconds

    G)   60 gtt/min = 1 gtt/s = 1 drip every second

    H)   20 gtt/min = 0.333 gtt/s = 5 drips every 15 seconds

    I)   100 gtt/min = 1.667 gtt/s = 15 drips every 25 seconds or 3 drips every 5 seconds

    J)   13.889 gtt/min = 0.2315 gtt/s = 0.926 drips every 4 seconds = 1 drip every 4 seconds

4   A)   0.135 gtt/s = 2.02 drips every 15 seconds = 2 drips every 15 seconds

    B)   0.2338 gtt/s = 3.97 drips every 19 seconds = 4 drips every 19 seconds

    C)   0.1667 gtt/s = 1 drip every 6 seconds

    D)   0.472 gtt/s = 9.92 drips every 21 seconds = 10 drips every 21 seconds

    E)   0.533 gtt/s = 10.1 drips every 19 seconds = 10 drips every 19 seconds

    F)   0.84 gtt/s = 5.04 drips every 6 seconds = 5 drips every 6 seconds

    G)   1.408 gtt/s = 7.04 drips every 5 seconds = 7 drips every 5 seconds

    H)   0.8468 gtt/s = 11.08 drips every 13 seconds = 11 drips every 13 seconds

I)   0.236 gtt/s = 4.01 drips every 17 seconds = 4 drips every 17 seconds

J)   0.463 gtt/s = 6.02 drips every 13 seconds = 6 drips every 13 seconds

5   A)   minimum rate = 40 mL/h; maximum rate = 120 mL/h

B)   minimum rate = 14 mL/h; maximum rate = 21 mL/h

C)   minimum rate = 86.4 mL/h; maximum rate = 259.2 mL/h

D)   minimum rate = 8.6 mL/h; maximum rate = 12.9 mL/h

E)   minimum rate = 30 mL/h; maximum rate = 90 mL/h

F)   minimum rate = 5 mL/h; maximum rate = 7.5 mL/h

G)   minimum rate = 75.5 mL/h; maximum rate = 226.4 mL/h

H)   minimum rate = 5.7 mL/h; maximum rate = 8.5 mL/h

I)   minimum rate = 40.2 mL/h; maximum rate = 120.7 mL/h

J)   minimum rate = 9.8 mL/h; maximum rate = 14.7 mL/h

6   A)   441 mL in 24 hours; 18.4 mL per hour

B)   267 mL in 24 hours; 11.1 mL per hour

C)   1797 mL in 24 hours; 74.9 mL per hour

D)   194 mL in 24 hours; 8.1 mL per hour

E)   817 mL in 24 hours; 34 mL per hour

F)   220 mL in 24 hours; 9.2 mL per hour

G)   1663 mL in 24 hours; 69.3 mL per hour

H)   287 mL in 24 hours; 12 mL per hour

7   A)   800 mL replace + 480 mL 24 hours maintenance = 1280 mL/24 hours, 53.3 mL/h, 0.889 mL/min, 13.3 gtt/min for this IV set calibration

B)   240 mL replace + 192 mL 24 hours maintenance = 432 mL/24 hours, 18 mL/h, 0.3 mL/min, 18 gtt/min for this IV set calibration

    C) 1200 mL replace + 960 mL 24 hours maintenance = 2160 mL/24 hours, 90 mL/h, 1.5 mL/min, 30 gtt/min for this IV set calibration

    D) 364 mL replace + 218 mL 24 hours maintenance = 582 mL/24 hours, 24.2 mL/h, 0.4 mL/min, 8 gtt/min for this IV set calibration

    E) 2745 mL replace + 1647 mL 24 hours maintenance = 4393 mL/24 hours, 183 mL/h, 3 mL/min, 30 gtt/min

    F) 239 mL replace + 115 mL 24 hours maintenance = 354 mL/24 hours, 14.7 mL/h, 0.25 mL/min, 15 gtt/min

    G) 2350 mL replace + 1128 mL 24 hours maintenance = 3478 mL/24 hours, 145 mL/h, 2.4 mL/min, 36 gtt/min

    H) 180 mL replace + 108 mL 24 hours maintenance = 288 mL/24 hours, 12 mL/h, 0.2 mL/min, 4 gtt/min

8 A) 3 hour 45 minute infusion ending at 6:55 p.m. or 18:55

    B) 4 hour infusion ending at 2:55 p.m. or 14:55

    C) 5 hour infusion ending at 6:35 p.m. or 18:35

    D) 9 hour infusion ending at 4:25 a.m. or 04:25 tomorrow morning

    E) 7 hour and 40 minute infusion ending at 7:25 a.m. or 07:25 tomorrow morning

    F) 4 hour and 40 minute infusion ending at 8:35 a.m. or 08:35

Chapter 10 Answers

1 A) 10

    B) 36

    C) 30

    D) 128

    E) 8

2 A) 1 part solute, 19 parts diluent, 20 parts final solution

    B) 1 part solute, 319 parts diluent, 320 parts final solution

C) 2 parts solute, 3 parts diluent, 5 parts total solution

D) 5 parts solute, 35 parts diluent, 40 parts total solution

E) 10 parts solute, 240 parts diluent, 250 parts total solution

3 A) 0.2 mg/mL

   B) 0.02% = 0.02 g/100 mL = 20 mg/100 mL = 0.2 mg/mL

   C) 0.2 g/L = 200 mg/L = 200 mg/1000 mL = 0.2 mg/mL

   D) 0.1875% = 0.1875 g/100 mL = 187.5 mg/100 mL = 1.875 mg/mL

   E) 0.005333 mg/mL

4 A) 60 mL of 12.5 mg/mL final solution; 45 mL of diluent was added

   B) 12.5 mL of 20 mg/mL final solution; 10 mL of diluent was added

   C) 125 mL of 10 mg/mL final solution; 75 mL of diluent was added

   D) 14 mL of 3.125 mg/mL final solution; 10.5 mL of diluent was added

   E) 6.4 mL of 1.875% final solution; 2.4 mL of diluent was added

5 A) 31.25 mL of original solution needed; 93.75 mL diluent needed

   B) 8 mL of original solution needed; 32 mL diluent added

   C) 25 mL of original solution needed; 75 mL diluent added

   D) 0.2 mL of original solution needed; 3.8 mL diluent added

   E) 125 mL of original solution needed; 125 mL of diluent added

   F) 150 mL of original solution needed; 350 mL of diluent added

   G) 16 mL of original solution needed; 84 mL of diluent added

   H) 3.125 mL of original solution needed; 21.875 mL of diluent added

   I) 1.25 mL of original solution needed; 248.75 mL of diluent added

J) 50 mL of original solution needed; 50 mL of diluent added

K) 125 mL of original solution needed; 75 mL of diluent added

L) 156.25 mL of original solution needed; 93.75 mL of diluent added

M) 60 mL of original solution needed; 60 mL of diluent added

6 A) final diluted solution is 22 mL with concentration of 9.1 mg/mL

B) 100 mL of concentrated disinfectant with 100 mL of diluent

C) 160 mL of 3% concentrated solution (3% = 30 mg/mL)

D) volume of the final solution is 160 mL and the volume of diluent is 150 mL

7 A) 1 : 10 = 10% solution; 62.5 mL of original solution plus 87.5 mL of diluent

B) 750 mg/mL = 75% solution; 1:2 = 1/2 = 0.5 = 50% solution; 6 mL of diluent and 18 mL of final diluted solution

C) 6% = 60 mg/mL; 300 mL of 80 mg/mL concentrated drug

D) 2% = 20 mg/mL or 480 mg/mL = 48%; 12.5 mL of concentrated drug and 287.5 mL of diluent

E) 5:8 = 5/8 = 0.625 = 62.5%; 375 mL of diluted 2% solution

Chapter 11 Answers

1 A) mean 8.73, median 9, mode 9, range 14

B) mean 36.8, median 38, mode 38, range 21

C) mean 1.35, median 1.38, mode 1.38, range 0.17

D) mean −0.1, median 0.25, mode 0.3, range 3.2 (2.4 below zero to 0.8 above zero)

E) mean 24.8, median 24.9, mode 22.3, range 15

2 A) 15.6 °C

B) 32.2 °C

C) 40.0 °C

D) 42.2 °C

E) −23 °C

F) 38.6 °C

G) 37.2 °C

H) 53.3 °C

I) 39.1 °C

J) 38.2 °C

3　A) 95 °F

B) 108 °F

C) 53.6 °F

D) 26.6 °F

E) 98.6 °F

F) 105 °F

G) −49 °F

H) 99.9 °F

I) 97.3 °F

J) 101 °F

4　A) 12

B) 25

C) 47 (−10 + 50 + 5 + 1 + 1)

D) 64 (50 + 10 − 1 + 5)

E) 93 (−10 + 100 + 1 + 1 + 1)

F) 129

G) 334

H) 1237

I) 1935 (1000 − 100 + 1000 + 10 + 10 + 10 + 5)

J) 1998 (1000 − 100 + 1000 − 10 + 100 + 5 + 1 + 1 + 1)

5   A) VIII

B) XXIII

C) XLV

D) CII

E) CCCXIX

F) CDLXXVII

G) DCCCXVI

H) MCCCXCIII

I) MCMXCIV

J) MMXIX

6   A) 8 + 115 = 123 = CXXIII

B) 15 + 42 = 57 = LVII

C) 95 − 24 = 71 = LXXI

D) 114 − 49 = 65 = LXV

E) 613 + 413 = 1023 = MXXIII

F) 99 + 101 + 74 = 274 = CCLXXIV

G) 2326 − 1919 = 407 = CDVII

H) 1052 − 501 = 551 = DLI

7   38 °C = 100.4 °F so the 100.9 °F is an increase in body temperature over the previous day.

Index

Medical Mathematics and Dosage Calculations for Veterinary Technicians, Third Edition. Robert Bill.
© 2019 John Wiley & Sons, Inc. Published 2019 by John Wiley & Sons, Inc.
Companion website: www.wiley.com/go/bill/calculations